UNLOCKED:
FROM PSYCH HOSPITAL
TO HIGHER SELF

UNLOCKED:
FROM PSYCH HOSPITAL TO HIGHER SELF

25 Keys to Recovering
from Depression, Anxiety,
or Bipolar Disorder

Emily Grossman

MA, CPRP

MEDIA

Note: a number of names in this book have been changed to protect confidentiality.

Published 2023 by Gildan Media LLC
aka G&D Media
www.GandDmedia.com

Front cover design by Tom McKeveny
Front cover photo by Jim Esposito

Designed by Meghan Day Healey of Story Horse, LLC.

Library of Congress Cataloging-in-Publication Data is available upon request

ISBN: 978-1-7225-0652-0

10 9 8 7 6 5 4 3 2 1

To my parents, Nina and Rich Grossman.
Let's be family in the next life too.

Contents

Prelude

Locked Up

I will never forget the helpless look on my parents' faces. It was 1996, and it was supposed to be my first semester of freshman year in college. As the large-framed orderly pulled me through the hall and behind the heavy doors, I screamed, "No, no, no, let me go home." Looking behind me, I could see Mom leaning on Dad's shoulder, crying, as he rubbed her back to console her. I flailed my arms and legs. I tried to break free of the orderly's strong grip and wrestled with him futilely until the heavy doors slammed shut and locked behind us with a hollow click.

That click represented more than doors locking: it separated me from not only my parents but from life as I had known it up to that point. I know a piece of me remained behind those heavy, gray metal doors, as if my soul had been left on the other side of them.

I tried to assess my surroundings through my tears and perceived everything as misshapen. The people roaming the halls aimlessly were distorted in much the way that a fun house mirror shrinks or stretches out objects depending upon the angle at which you look at them. My tears made everything fuzzy and out of focus. My head throbbed, my throat was scratchy from screaming, and I was physically exhausted from the intense events of the day.

I wiped my eyes enough to notice the cold, pale blue walls, which I would learn later were a mental institution cliché. Some psychologist somewhere had believed light blue to be a calming color, so most of these psych wards were painted in this shade, which I grew to detest. Like bank tellers, nurses sat motionlessly behind a thick glass window with a hole on the bottom for speaking through. They were staring at the patients walking by, watching us as if we were fish in an aquarium. Even with the bright fluorescent lights, the place felt totally dark.

On the walls were posters with trite sayings like "One day at a time" and "Easy does it." I felt deeply resentful of the people who decided to hang such posters on the wall. It's easy for them to give advice when they aren't held against their will in a psych ward.

"C'mon in, and let's get some linens for your bed," the orderly said, trying to be warm and nonjudgmental. But let's be real: he was judging. My identity from that moment on was going to be forever changed. This orderly would be the first to greet me not as Emily Grossman, eighteen-year-old Emory University freshman with all the promise in the world, but as Emily Grossman, the eighteen-year-old mental patient. It was as if by handing me those starchy white sheets, this man was handing me my future, one that looked extremely bleak.

Introduction

B ooks about personal transformation often use the metaphor of a phoenix rising from the ashes to describe the journey. For those of you unfamiliar with this metaphor, it implies that out of the fires of misfortune, a new and better self emerges. While I find this interesting, I more like to liken my own personal journey to an old fable that I've heard through my years of Buddhist practice. In this fable, the Buddha meets a young man who is going around begging for food. When the beggar is not looking, the Buddha sews a precious jewel into his robe. The beggar goes on with his life begging. When the beggar sees the Buddha again, he is an old man. The Buddha is surprised to find him still begging and his robe still tattered. The beggar had spent his lifetime looking outside of himself to survive when he had all the riches of the world in his possession already; he just didn't realize it.

For as long as I can remember, I struggled to find my own inner riches externally while putting a great deal of pressure on myself. On my tenth birthday, which I had labeled "The Big 1-0," I told my father that I was excited to get older because it meant that I would be closer to being perfect—because adults are perfect. Yikes!

Growing up, I was plagued by low self-esteem and little belief that I could do well in life. I didn't believe in my internal strength, and I certainly didn't believe in the divinity that lies within me. It was a difficult struggle as I tried to overcompensate in many ways, not the least of which was my perfectionism.

True to perfectionistic form, when I was first diagnosed with bipolar disorder in 1996, I was ready to devote my whole self to finding a cure. I remember telling my friends in my dorm at Emory that I was going to leave school to tour around with my parents and find the most effective (read: perfect) treatment for what was ailing me. My parents had a different plan: to get me stable and get me back to school as soon as possible. Neither plan seemed to be effective, and as I will detail shorty, I was soon thrust into a complicated web of mental health treatment that ultimately went nowhere fast.

This book is the culmination of the knowledge that I've amassed in two-plus decades since my diagnosis and my subsequent recovery. It contains a powerful roadmap to help you discover *your* inner riches—the very ones that you need to overcome a behavioral health struggle. I want it to be the book that I needed back then—one that not only tells my story but helps you to understand what recovery from mental illness can look like and how to get there. If you apply the lessons that I offer, you can learn how not only to overcome a mental health challenge but to have a jumping-off point through which you can grow spiritually.

This book is about how to weave all the complex moving parts required for recovery into a beautiful tapestry of strategies that put you in the driver's seat to recovery. I would also like to open a window to your Higher Self or Higher Power (whichever idea you resonate with more).

There are a few important things to know about the structure of the book before you proceed. It is organized chronologically, but each vignette that I put in the book is followed by a "lesson learned" section in which I reveal a key that unlocked me from the seeming jail sentence that was mental illness. I invite you to use whatever metaphor for the Divine that feels most appropriate for you. Whether you or a loved one are struggling with a mental illness or you just want to read a story that will inspire you, I have tried to outline, through many vignettes, the steps that I took to reach my Higher Self.

As stated earlier, this book does have a deeply spiritual component. I could not have overcome my own struggles were it not for spirituality. Although I want this book to be accessible to all, it is written from a Buddhist lens, because that is my spiritual practice. I am not doing this to proselytize. I deeply respect and value many different spiritual practices, but Buddhism is the one that I know intimately enough to speak about how it has helped me to transform my life. Still, to be more inclusive, I've referred to a Higher Power in this book. Every time I am speaking about a Higher

Power, I have capitalized the words so that they will stand out to you, as well as to show deep respect for the forces that guide the Universe.

The next thing I'd like to explain is the idea of mental health recovery. I realize that this is a loaded concept, because there is a popular belief that mental illness is the kind of thing that you live with forever. I assure you that I have found this to be far from true. I am a living example that people can get well from mental illnesses such as bipolar disorder. And by recovery, I mean the resolution of symptoms. I do not have the symptoms of my mental illness that I had thirteen years ago, which included mania, depression, psychosis, and chronic suicidal ideation. After using the keys in this book, I entered a period of what I would describe not as stability—which implies that you can be destabilized at any time—but as deep inner serenity, where I live a highly successful, virtually symptom-free life. I still have highs and lows and intense emotions in life, and I have to work consistently, in fact daily, at managing my mental health, particularly anxiety. But I'm grateful to say that my baseline is one of inner calm and tranquility.

While recovery from mental illness and its meaning have been hotly debated, neuroscience has discovered that brains are not static, as was once believed, but highly plastic. The neurotransmitters in one's brain can change, and new pathways can be formed that change one's life experience. Without getting too deeply into the science of it, this is what I believe has happened to my own brain in over two decades of doing the spiritual work that I will describe in this book.

I *know* that I do not have the same brain because my bipolar brain at its worst could barely use an ATM machine—too much inner preoccupation, too much psychosis, and too many steps to retrieve my money. Obviously a lot has changed since then, and I'm thrilled and eager to impart what I've learned in the chapters that follow. In sum, I've learned the complex set of moving parts that manage the machine that is recovery. It's not just therapy and medication that have placed me on this path, although these have been critical parts of my journey, and I still am involved with both.

Before I reveal too much about the antidote to my ills, I would like to give you a brief overview of my story. After that, we will go on to the vignettes so that you can dig into the keys to overcoming your own struggles and living a recovered life. The promise of this book is not just that you can recover by following the keys, but that you can thrive and become a deeply connected spiritual being. Sound too good to be true? Well, hang with me—there's much to explain and much to learn.

To get us started, what you should know about young Emily (and what I've alluded to earlier) is that I had all the traits of your typical Type A personality. I loved making lists of tasks that I had to complete and got a great deal of satisfaction from checking them off, using the special line that I had written next to the task where the check mark belonged. A self-improvement junkie, I pored over the articles in my teenybopper magazines with titles like "Use This Mask for Perfect Skin" or "Ten Exercises for Your Best Body Now." I also remember being in high school and listening to the audio recording of Stephen Covey's *Seven Habits of Highly Effective*

People in my car while driving to and from the gym, while many of my peers were listening to Led Zeppelin, The Doors, and Phish.

Putting this much pressure on myself created a sort of dual life. On the one hand, I had a very successful academic experience in grammar and high school. I also had a full social life in high school, with many friends, and was rarely without a boyfriend. As I gather from reports from my peers, it seemed to them that I had it all together, and that's what I wanted them to think. But keeping up this appearance was soul-crushing, and by junior year of high school, I found myself not only anxious and depressed but contemplating suicide for the first time, although I told no one.

By the time I got to Emory University, I brought with me a fractured self. The first few months of my geographic cure of getting far from my New Jersey home worked beautifully, and I fell in love with school. However, soon the novelty wore off, and I was stuck back with my dual existence—seemingly perfect on the outside (at least that's what I tried to project) while haunted by demons on the inside. Although it was traumatic, it really came as no surprise to me when I had to leave Emory for mental health treatment. I couldn't keep up the lie anymore, and I didn't want to. It was too exhausting.

Still, perfectionism clung to me even as I boarded the plane from Atlanta to Newark, New Jersey. I told my friends that I was leaving school in search of the perfect cure for my illness. In reality, I was deeply ashamed and humiliated that I had to leave school and felt that I had ruined my life. I had worked hard to get into Emory, and I felt lost without my identity as a college student, and deeply suicidal as a result.

It was not until I was sitting on my hospital bed in Car-rier Clinic in Belle Mead, New Jersey, after being hospitalized for suicidal thoughts that I realized that there was no perfect solution. It turned out that I had a family history of mental illness on my father's side. I felt boxed in and doomed to follow in the footsteps of some of my relatives, which included at best social isolation, and at worst incarceration.

There is something about being labeled bipolar, as I had been by that point. It takes away not only one's sense of confi-dence but also one's humanity. Once I had a diagnosis, people stopped understanding me as Emily Grossman and started thinking of me as a mental patient. And I certainly followed suit. Any self-esteem that I had left was stripped away and replaced by a deep sense of being damaged goods.

While I did return to college the following fall, this time at Rutgers University, the idea that I was damaged took me to some dark places, especially into an emotionally and verbally abusive relationship that would continue on and off for nearly a decade.

Aside from this unfortunate turn of events, I met a new master in college, which took the form of psychosis. Once I was deeply delusional, seeing and hearing things that were not there, all bets were off. I went into and out of the psychiat-ric hospital twelve times. I lost most of my friends in my senior year of college, alienated roommates, and graduated by the skin of my delusional teeth.

Graduating was extremely anticlimactic for me. It was expected that I would finish school, and although I worked hard writing papers while experiencing delusions and hal-lucinations, once I graduated, I became a shell of my former self. I didn't have the structure of school to organize my life around. All I knew how to do was be a student.

And there were many losses at the end of college. My grandmother died about a week before I graduated, but I had no time to grieve, as I was writing papers. My boyfriend and I broke up, which, while positive for both of us, was also deeply troubling at the time because, as abusive as he was, he was also my caretaker. This may seem like an odd dichotomy, but one thing that I learned through treatment was dialectical thinking—that two opposites can be true at the same exact time. At the time, I only knew that it was a total mind-&c%#@.

I set out to get a job, but along with my other diagnoses, I experienced a severe case of posttraumatic stress disorder: I was stammering my words when I spoke, like a shell-shocked veteran. Because of this, I was not exactly seen as the ideal candidate for any job that I interviewed for, even though my résumé and GPA were desirable. Additionally, by that time, I had been nearly institutionalized in a state hospital. The hospital had become such a part of me that I had few adult living skills. Yes, I did my own laundry and cooked a bit, but working, paying bills, and finding a place to live were just not in my wheelhouse at that point.

They often say that when a person has been in and out of a mental hospital as many times as I had, the hospital gets inside of them, and institutionalization becomes hard to shake. That is how people become mental patients: it's not the illnesses that make them that way, but the helplessness created by the system in which they are treated. This was the state that I found myself in in 2002, after narrowly escaping a life sentence at Trenton State Psychiatric Hospital. I had nowhere to live, nowhere to work, and no one to love (at least not romantically). I also had very few friends left.

Fortunately, my war-torn parents, who were beaten down by years of my unrelenting crises, did find me a placement in a living situation called "supported housing," where I was living with other mentally ill women, all schizophrenic, and mostly above the age of sixty. It was a low bottom for me as I watched all my friends from college get exciting jobs in Manhattan and move to Hoboken or Jersey City. It was also a supreme motivator.

Through sheer will, I began to pick myself back up again and start working—first just filing papers part-time in a law office where one of my only remaining college friends was working. It was a boring and thankless job, and one that I lost very quickly, but at least it gave me some structure while I tried to find something more permanent. This was followed by my first permanent full-time job, which was working as a supervisor for tutors at a tutoring center—another job that I had for under a year. But, little by little, I was starting to join the land of the living again. While I wasn't exactly thriving in mainstream society, I was no longer fully on the fringes. I moved to Belmar, New Jersey (think the show *The Jersey Shore*), with some women my age. Again, while the situation was tenuous, it was certainly better than my previous living situation. From there I strung together about a year of work in education, first as a substitute teacher, and then as an admin and tutor at an SAT test prep center. I ended up keeping this job only for another nine months, but I knew one thing for certain—I wanted to become a "great educator," whatever that meant.

During my illness, I kept on hearing a message that told me that I was meant to "make a difference in the world." I didn't know how, but I remembered being a young girl, and loving to play school with all my dolls and Barbies. I even taught all my lessons from the day at school in order to study for my classes (an idea that I came up with on my own). This continued through college.

I'm not sure what gave me the confidence to apply for a graduate program at Columbia University's Teachers College, but I picked up the tattered and battered pieces of myself and filled out that application. Then, miraculously, I was accepted—and terrified.

The people I loved and trusted the most kept advising me not to go: it was expensive, and I couldn't keep a job. I'd have to take out student loans, and I was in debt. I couldn't take care of myself, let alone a group of students. It was in Manhattan, and I knew nothing about navigating the city.

However, something told me it was the right choice. So after deferring for a year, deliberating, and not getting anywhere, I decided to go. I know now that every dollar that I spent there was worth it because it powerfully kick-started my first glimpses of recovery. Also, within the first few months of graduate school, I encountered the Buddhist practice that would help me to rebuild and recreate my life.

We know now that when one is coming out of psychosis for the amount of time that I experienced it, there is often some loss of executive functioning. I was definitely experiencing that when I went to school. It can be reversed through something called *cognitive remediation*. But I didn't know that at the time, nor did I have that treatment. What I did have was the mediation practice of chanting the Buddhist mantra that I believe rebuilt my brain and helped me to begin to rebuild my life.

When I began chanting, I wasn't expecting much. I didn't even like doing it at first; I found it arduous and joyless. But I loved the philosophy that my dear friend Gonzalo was teaching me about. This philosophy, along with the chanting, would help me to manifest a life beyond anything I could ever have imagined.

There were five important things on my list to manifest that year, and through universal forces, they all started to come true. These things included getting a job near Hoboken, getting a car, finding an apartment in Hoboken, teaching sixth or seventh grade, and overcoming my symptoms of mental illness. While these needs were quite practical, the series of synchronicities that enabled me to manifest each one (which I will get into later) convinced me that there was something to this practice.

After graduate school, I began teaching seventh grade in a school near Hoboken. While I loved the kids and the job very much, by my tenure year I was experiencing a bit of a relapse in the form of depression. Although my practice had helped me to overcome my symptoms of mental illness, I would learn that I had to do some more "human revolution," transforming something deep within myself, before the symptoms would be permanently eradicated. Although I believe that the chanting kept them from getting much worse, I did have to be hospitalized again for the last time.

In addition to my depression, during that time I noticed that a lot of my students were coming to me with their own mental health struggles. While I was concerned and committed to wanting to help them, the administration told me to leave that to the school guidance counselor and social worker. In my tenure year, I simultaneously decided to change careers and was dismissed from my teaching position.

In the meantime, what happened to my Buddhist practice? I was chanting a lot less. But the most important thing to understand is that my practice doesn't prevent the inevitable ups and downs of life. It simply provides a tool so that when these inevitable lows happen, one can turn poison into medicine.

After being dismissed in March, I knew I wanted to get into mental health. But taking out yet another big loan to become a social worker just wasn't feasible. After some research, I found a program that would train me to coach people who had been struggling with behavioral health challenges, based on my own experience of living with and working to overcome my own challenges. This was called being a "peer provider."

I lost the teaching job in March, but thanks to my prayers, I was able to find a peer provider job by April. I had also convinced my administration to pay me out for the rest of the teaching year, which they agreed to do, so I found myself with two salaries at that point. I *know* that I couldn't have done this without the help of my prayers.

Working as a peer provider was extremely rewarding. I began working for a community mental health center in New Jersey, coaching adults on their recoveries. I ran groups and worked with people individually. It was extremely rewarding, and it was where I was meant to be at that time. In addition, my recovery started to improve. My confidence started to return, and I knew that while helping others, I was also helping myself to move on.

I worked in two roles as a peer provider, and in the second, I was helping people with behavioral health challenges to find employment. During this time, my recovery was starting to take off, and I saw many others recover with my support. I even helped one woman to get a job making double what I was making at the time and provided her with the support to be successful on that job.

While I was doing all of this, a new dream grew in my heart: I wanted to combine my passion for educating with my passion for mental health recovery. I chanted deeply about this and manifested my first job working in New York City and Long Island as a trainer of mental health professionals. This was my true calling.

For the last decade, I have been working in training in different roles. Currently I work as a director of a training institute at a behavioral health nonprofit in Manhattan. I love the role, and I've had the opportunity to train thousands of behavioral health providers as well as build a training institute from the ground up, which has been deeply satisfying.

Along the way, there have been many twists and turns, which the rest of this book will detail, but with each one, my recovery and my spiritual practice have grown deeper and stronger. My life has become richer, more solid, and most importantly, much happier. The rest of this book is meant to give you a more detailed sense of what it was like for me, how I used spirituality to transform my life, and what things are like now.

And so, my dear reader, we are about to embark upon a journey towards self-transformation together. As with any journey, there will be highs and lows, but I can promise you that if you stay the course, you hold in your hands right now an opportunity to look deeply within, see what has you stuck, and make the changes necessary to live your best life. We have only a short time in this life, so I implore you to get started. A rich life awaits you on the other side of these pages. In the words of the great Jewish teacher Hillel, "If not now, when?"

Follow Your Bliss

I had a lot on my mind as a sophomore at Marlboro High School in 1992. Ah, Marlboro. This town, located just one hour southwest of New York City, was once all farmland and clay. The "marl" in Marlboro is a clay that can be found in its soil. The Native Americans used it to make clay pots and such (at least that's what Ms. Breen told us in third grade).

Growing up in Marlboro was wonderful in many ways. It was a suburb of New York City, so very often my parents or friends and I would hop on a train and go into the city. The sprawling farmland was sold and turned into the kind of soccer fields that any soccer mom would adore. The school district was highly regarded, and in an upper-middle class suburb—none of my friends ever had to deal with the pain of poverty or starvation.

However, there was something in the air in Marlboro—let's for now call it "friendly competition." There were *expecta-*

tions, which started among the parents, but dripped down to the kids like water in a leaky faucet. Conversations amongst parents when I was young would go something like this: "I would have let David come over to play today, but he's so busy, what with travel soccer, his homework for the gifted and talented program, and gymnastics competition that he couldn't possibly have time." To this, the other mother would respond, "Well, that's OK. My son was busy too: he was working on his science fair project—which he, by the way, got an A+ on—and taking his concert piano lessons, so he couldn't have had a friend over anyway."

This competition continued throughout my youth and into my adolescence. The conversation became different, but the main messages were still the same. How come my father, who, bless his heart, traveled back and forth to New York City every day with many of the other Marlboro fathers, could tell me by the time he got home at night exactly what my schoolmates' SAT scores were, where they were going to college, and what they were majoring in? Believe me: it wasn't because he was interested. It was because the competition conversation continued from Marlboro to New York City, and then all the way back home.

As I said before, there were *expectations* in Marlboro. Not from my parents, but from the general masses—expectations about how well one did in school, how one dressed, the kind of car one drove, the extracurricular activities that one was involved in. Being someone who always wanted to be her best self, I certainly got wrapped up in all of this. Part of it was just trying to fit in. Part of it was that I am competitive by nature. But I put so much pressure on myself to fit the Marlboro mold. I had to look, dress, achieve, and generally fit in with the high standards set by many parents and absorbed by their children.

So by sophomore year, I had a lot on my mind. I was in an advanced business program and taking many of the school's AP and honors classes at the same time. I also was keenly aware, every time I passed by the school's mirrored hallways, that I had to maintain my appearance. I scoured fashion magazines weekly in the hopes that I would arrive at school looking as if I had just walked off their pages. Then there was cheerleading. I was on the junior varsity team, and just *had* to make varsity by my junior year. Also on my mind: SATs, boys, parties, and did I mention boys?

In the midst of all of this, there was one oasis—Mrs. Collin's class. Mrs. Collins was an English teacher, often seen in her iconic preppy walking shorts. She always had a twinkle in her eye and love for her students in her heart. Yet she was also tough when she needed to be—especially when grading our papers. She knew how to set the bar just high enough that one had to take a leap to reach it, but not so high that one would become frustrated by an inability to reach the goal. We all loved her. And we all *worked* in her class. I loved the way she read Shakespeare to us, emphasizing the parts that meant the most to her and teaching us critical analytical skills simultaneously. She taught me to think in this way through her sheer skill and talent as a teacher.

About midway through the year, Mrs. Collins introduced us to the works of Joseph Campbell. Campbell, an author and a professor at Sarah Lawrence College, studied myths and looked for commonalities between them. During this unit on

Campbell, a moment happened which would alter the course of my life, though I did not know it at the time.

That day, Mrs. Collins had navy blue and green plaid walking shorts, with navy tights, loafers, and a navy turtleneck. She bounced into the room with the energy of someone half her age, which was no different than usual. Then she picked up a piece of chalk and wrote this on the board: "I say, follow your bliss, and don't be afraid, and the Universe will open doors where you didn't know they were going to be."

"What does this quote by Campbell mean to you?" Mrs. Collins asked, her eyes sparkling.

I don't remember if I raised my hand to answer the question, but I instantly knew the meaning. I had been living my life in a fear-based way, trying to please everyone but myself, and thinking that this was success. But here was Mrs. Collins reassuring me that if I followed the thing that made me most happy, I would be supported by the Universe. I felt every muscle in my ninety-pound, five-foot-three-inch body instantly relax. I believed Campbell, but more than that, I believed and trusted Mrs. Collins.

I wish I could say that this changed me right away, but it didn't. There were too many pressures in high school, and I was still too set on fitting in to change my ways. But I internalized that message and have used it at many pivotal moments. When someone has bipolar disorder with a tendency towards suicidal thoughts, they must be aware of what makes them happy and follow their bliss. The alternative can be death. I know that this may sound dramatic, but it is not.

Luckily, suicidal thoughts have been my "true north": my way of knowing if the path that I'm on in life is working or isn't. And following my bliss has worked every time. There have been some difficult decisions. I've made some sharp turns in my career. But today I'm extremely happy, and I know that it's because when I felt stuck, I identified my bliss at every turn.

How do you know when you are following your bliss? It's different for everyone, but I'll try to describe how it feels to me. My body gives me signals when I'm on the right track, and so does the Higher Mind. When I'm following my bliss, my solar plexus, the area of the body at the middle of the chest, feels lighter. It's almost as if I can feel my heart start to flutter with excitement. I feel tingly in my fingers and feet. I am fully focused in the moment, so much so that as I was writing this afternoon (which is part of my bliss), someone came by and said, "Emily, you are not just working at your computer; it looks like your computer has swallowed you whole—like you are inside of it."

When I'm following my bliss, I don't feel any resistance from the Universe. I feel the opposite of stuck. I get things done at lightning speed. I feel I'm being inspired by the Divine Energy. It's as if whatever I'm working on is coming through me, and I am just the channel through which it will be delivered. My thoughts are clear and sharp. My energy is high, and I can concentrate for long stretches of time.

Following your bliss is critical if you want to come to your Highest Self. When you are basing your life choices on your bliss, you are following the path that you were meant to follow. That's why there is no resistance. When you continue on this path, you don't have to work so hard at making money. The resources you need, money included, are delivered by Spirit.

The hard part is trusting the Universe. But you will be given signs from Grace about whether you are on the right path. Just this past weekend, I felt stuck until I received a Tarot reading that helped me to become clear about my next career goals. I looked outside my window and there was a big sign written in chalk on the sidewalk. Its message: "Trust the process." Since I am usually impatient with myself about achieving goals, this was the perfect message for that day. Please don't overlook these signs. They are there for a reason.

Sell It

It's the spring of 1992. I walk out onto the stage, behind Hallie and Nikki, in pitch-black, my stomach swirling with a combination of anxiety and adrenaline. I can barely see the tape marks on the ground telling me where to stand, but I feel around for the X with my foot, and eventually I hit it. I must be very careful of where I stand, because one of the other girls who stands behind me has a mother who asked me not to block her. I pose with my back to the audience, leaning on my left leg, with my left hand on my hip. I am looking over my right shoulder, and my right hand is on the tip of my black cowboy hat. The lights come up, and the girls in the balcony— other dancers—start shouting and whistling, "Shake it, girls," and one of them screams in support.

In that split second before the music starts, I squeeze my lips together hard, trying to keep my serious face, as instructed by our teacher, George Warren. George, a man of about forty-five with an incredible skill for working with teenage girls, has worked hard preparing us for this day. I think of the words he always says to us in rehearsal: "Come on—sell it!"

The music comes on, and I begin to move. *"Desperado, why don't you come to your senses?"* The first part of the dance is lyrical, meaning that it's supposed to be danced slowly and emotionally. I love this part. I do an arabesque turn and start to really feel it. I forget about the fact that Kevin, a guy from high school, is sitting right in the front row with his family, and my ego wants to impress him and the other guys from my school who are there.

Soon the music changes to something more hip-hop and fast-paced, and you can not only hear the bass from the stage, you can feel it in your body. The tassels on my cowgirl costume are whirling through the air as I move through this section of the routine. I feel my adrenaline and anxiety return as we come towards the hardest part of the routine. Hallie, Nikki, and I take center stage. It's time for the quadruple pirouette turn. This is a move that requires not only balance but momentum, flexibility, and strength. I come directly into the moment—so much so that I can't even feel my body or see the crowd. It's just my soul out there. I *pas de bourrée* and then plant my foot. I don't allow any negativity to enter my mind. I place all the weight on that foot, and go up on my tippy-toe. The other leg rises up, so that my body looks as if my legs are making the number four. I swing around, whipping my head each time. I stay on my tiptoes, and I make it around four times. Victory! The crowd applauds loudly, and whistles can be heard. I feel incredibly proud, and in the moment, and I finish the routine with pure joy.

I get backstage, and George is standing there and gives me a big hug. "Wow!" he says. "You girls really sold it. Congratulations." I smile triumphantly and run to my next costume change full of pride.

The next key to becoming your Higher Self is to sell it. In dance, *selling it* means giving it your very best effort and giving an encore-worthy performance. This is a lot of pressure. Because I danced from the time I was three years old, I had some level of comfort on the stage by the time I was a teenager, but every time you go out before an audience, you are a beginner: every performance is new, and you only have one shot to woo your audience. There isn't a do-over in the live performing arts. Because of this, a high level of concentration is needed to nail a performance. During my years as a competitive dancer, I experimented with many different ways to make sure that I did just that. In the beginning of competitions, I was very nervous. Often the anxiety would get in the way, and I'd make mistakes. Only later would I realize what I was doing wrong: I was dancing with my ego instead of my heart.

What's the difference? When you are doing something with your ego, many times you are thinking, "I must do this perfectly to impress my boss," or "I have to give my best interview so that I get the job." Don't get me wrong: it's good to want to be your best. But you can't truly sell it, you can't perform at the highest level while being up in your ego and trying to impress people. Ego cuts us off from the Divine—the Higher Power that helps us to be our best. Doing something with your heart connects you to the Law That Guides All Things, which can help you give your best "performances."

So, you may ask, how do I connect to my heart and Spirit when I'm so anxious? The answer is twofold. First, be present. The present moment is where deep concentration can happen. Being present means getting out of one's way for long enough to let the sunlight of the Spirit come in. When your mind is in the past, you are probably reviewing things that you regret and beating yourself up. When your mind is in the future, you are probably worried about something that is going to happen. Neither mind state leads to selling it.

When our minds feel negative emotions, including anxiety, they often want to escape. So they start to think, usually about the past or future. Escaping this way disconnects us from our heart and Higher Power and prevents us from giving our best. You've heard the expression, "He's all up in his head"? It means you are thinking so much that you cannot perform at your best.

The second part of connecting to one's heart is to be of service. When I am thinking about giving a stellar performance, I'm not thinking about how my actions are affecting and hopefully helping others. By contrast, thinking from the perspective of service is a surefire way to get out of one's ego and work from the heart.

Here's how this looks in my life: I give lectures about my recovery from mental illness to a wide variety of audiences. I rarely know ahead of time who will be there. Yet I only have one shot at impressing the audience and connecting with them. When I'm up in my ego, trying to impress people, I am not my sharpest. I don't feed off the audience well; I'm not able to read the room. But when I stay in the moment and think of serving others—the mental health providers that I'm training and the clients who will ultimately receive their services—I'm agile enough to think on my feet and monitor my audience's reactions. This is when the magic happens. And the magic is that my Higher Power is working through me. I'm speaking from my heart, not from ego.

To get myself to this place, before I speak, I pray. I say to the Universe, "I will touch at least one person in the room today and inspire them that recovery is possible." When I reconnect myself to my mission and purpose, the process becomes not about me but about using my talents to serve the world and the Higher Mind. I am no longer hung up on the results and enjoy the process more. My true self comes out, and I can truly make an impact with my words. Then I can *sell it*.

⚷ ⎯⎯ Key 3

Find Your People

It was August 1996, and I was at Emory University, hav-ing a blast. Emory, a private university located in the heart of Atlanta, was physically stunning. The buildings were all white, and there were red and yellow tulips in beds, which really popped against the white buildings.

I had just come back from a whitewater rafting and camp-ing trip as part of freshman orientation. On the trip, I had made several friends and even started seeing a cute freshman named Joel. I was in all my glory. I also was doing great in my classes. My high-school career had been so rigorous academ-ically that I emerged a great student, and I found college no harder than my high-school classes.

Emotionally, I was on a high. I was also extremely social. Life felt perfect. In fact I was worried because I thought that it was a bit too perfect, and this thought was eerily prophetic.

In the beginning of October, it was my eighteenth birthday. I rounded up about eleven of my friends, and we went out to a bar/restaurant. It was a place downtown in Buckhead that was known for purposely having rude service as a prank. I thought it was hysterical, as did most of the friends who came along. We all were big binge drinkers and were partying up a storm. I couldn't have had a better night.

The next morning, when I woke up, I instantly felt it. It was wave after wave of sheer panic. I thought I was dying. I lay beneath my sheets shuddering and just couldn't get out of bed. It was a weekday, and I had to go to class, but I just couldn't.

The weekend before, a few of my friends and I had gone to see the movie *Trainspotting*, which was about a group of friends who used heroin. There was a scene in which one of the character's mothers locked him in a room and took away his heroin in an attempt to detox him. It showed the sheer agony that he was going through—sweating, screaming, and pulling his hair out. It also showed the room spinning around faster and faster. This scene is the closest that I can come to describing my experience that morning.

In deep despair and fear, I called my mother in New Jersey.

"M-m-mom," I said, barely able to get her name out.

"Honey," Mom said, "are you OK?"

"No, mom, I'm n-n-n-not. I don't know what's happening to me, but I feel like I'm dying."

"Have you seen anyone, honey? Like a doctor?" Mom said, sounding a bit concerned.

"No, mom, I c-c-can't. I'm stuck in my bed," I said.

"Em, what do you mean?" Mom said in a stern voice. "You need either to get up and go to the doctor or go to class. I mean, you can't miss class."

But I just couldn't do it. I stayed in my room all day and for a few days after.

Finally I crawled out of bed and thought of where I could go. My body was weak from not eating and barely drinking. The safest, most grounded friend I had was Mustafa, whom we all called "Moose." I tried to comb my hair, crawled to the elevator, and took it up one floor to Moose's room. Luckily, he was there, sitting on his bed, eating some food that his mom had brought down for him. He could tell immediately that something was seriously wrong.

"Ems," he said, "what brought this on?" I climbed into his bed and stuffed my head into his pillow. The sheets on his bed were checkered navy and white, and they smelled good. He must have just washed them.

"I-I-I don't know," I said, stuttering. "I'm afraid, though."

"Maybe you are having some kind of breakdown, Ems. My aunt and uncle are psychiatrists, and I've heard about this. You should go to the counseling center," he said, cuddling up next to me.

Although I was dating Joel, Moose and I also had a special connection. We were the best of friends at that time, and I would often cuddle with him. I was young, and I didn't know my boundaries with men. So cuddle with Moose I did. It was what I needed.

Soon, though, Moose had to go to class. "Let me help you get to the counseling center," he said and pulled me out of his bed. He practically had to carry me there. As I walked into the counseling center, I knew that it was where I should be. I hugged Moose goodbye and walked in.

The third key to becoming your Higher Self is to know who your people are—using your senses to figure out whom you can trust. I was always pretty good with this, but going through the struggles that I went through, I would get much better.

Amassing friends and supporters is extremely important for getting through difficult times. During my experience, I would find that the most important thing that I could do was find love and friendship.

E. M. Forster said, "Only connect." This is so true. Even though there were times that I was experiencing an isolating disease, I found that I was able to stay afloat because I was connected to my friends and loved ones.

Connecting is a skill. It takes time, perseverance, and even work. It takes reaching out to people and letting them know what is going on in your life, and equally, being there to support them through whatever is going on in theirs.

My illness could have ravaged me completely. It could have taken me out of life for good or delivered me into an institution for life. Yet my social skills, and finding my people wherever I went, kept me from both outcomes. I knew I had love and was loved, so I didn't want to end my life and hurt the people I was connected to. I also used my ability to connect to people to get out of situations like being institutionalized. People skills and connection were truly my best asset.

Regardless of what you are going through, I encourage you to follow Forster's words and never forget to connect with others. Find your people, and once you develop trusting, loving relationships with them, keep them close. Love is the answer to all ills in life. Of this I am convinced.

Find HP: Part 1

People often grapple with spirituality for a lifetime. This has not been my path. From a young age, I felt deeply connected to something, and for many years of my life, I was looking to give it a name.

By the time I was eighteen, in the spring of 1997, I had been hospitalized twice for depression and anxiety and finally diagnosed with bipolar II disorder. In the hospital, I felt that God was punishing me. I felt I was a bad person, and that was why I was put there in the first place.

Looking at God as someone that punishes and rewards people was not a stretch, given my upbringing. I was raised Jewish, and the Old Testament God often *did* do that. He was not even above asking Abraham to sacrifice his son Isaac to show his devotion. I sought out several rabbis to try and understand what was happening to me, but none of them seemed to have enough of a grasp on mental illness to help me.

After I was released from my second hospitalization at age eighteen, I came home traumatized, disillusioned, and dejected. It had been decided that I could not return to Emory University, a place that represented every success that I had achieved up until that point. I would have to transfer to Rutgers, because it was closer to my doctors. I would start in the fall. It was January at this point, so I was left with a lot of unstructured time and a deep feeling of self-loathing.

In order to cope with having a daughter newly diagnosed with mental illness, my mother began to do a lot of spiritual reading. She too practiced Judaism but was very open-minded. In 1996, a ton of New Age books had come onto the market and were becoming popular. Mom read many of them. Books such as James Redfield's *Celestine Prophecy* and Deepak Chopra's *Seven Spiritual Laws of Success* could often be found strewn on the multicolored pastel comforter on the bed in her room. I would read with her.

I remember the first time that I read *The Seven Spiritual Laws of Success*. As I stared at the tan book jacket, I felt an energy that stilled my melancholy. I began reading: "Although this book is titled *The Seven Spiritual Laws of Success*, it could also be called *The Seven Spiritual Laws of Life*, because these are the same keys that nature uses to create everything in material existence—everything we can see, hear, smell, taste, or touch."

I was instantly hooked. The book, which talks about the greater laws of the Universe, was the perfect elixir for my illness of the spirit. It really lifted me. After reading the book in one day, I felt electricity racing through my body. I was not just inspired, I was temporarily transformed. Immediately I prayed to the God of the Old Testament.

"God," I said, "I am not finding what I need to understand the complexity of my mental health situation through Judaism. I am looking for a practice or religion like the one that I am reading about in this book." Little did I know that later my prayers would truly be answered.

The next key to restoring your mental health is to find your HP—your Higher Power, whether you see that as God, Universe, Source, or something else.

Coming across those books when I was feeling so lost and desperate was a major step in my healing. It reminded me of my HP. That didn't make the rest of my journey easy or fun, but it did make it possible.

In the Buddhist tradition that I am a part of, Nichiren Buddhism, the Higher Power is known as the Mystic Law. It's called "mystic" because it's beyond human comprehension. I think that at this stage in my journey, that was the best way to describe it. I deeply wanted to understand who or what my Higher Power was, but I had no real concept of one that made sense to me. I just couldn't wrap my head around who or what this power was. So at this time, while I was pretty angry with the God of my Jewish faith, I called my Higher Power the Universe. I look at this name as kind of a placeholder for something that admittedly I still don't fully comprehend in its entirety.

Yet I knew that I needed to believe that there was some benevolent force that just might have my back, and this was as far as I took it at the time. I will describe the evolution of my sense of a Higher Power later, but for now, I just want to say that if you don't have a Higher Power that you believe in, it's OK. Start simply. Some people begin by sitting in nature and make that their Higher Power. In my Buddhist practice, it's not even a power outside of oneself, but the Mystic Law: a power that is mostly within, like the Higher Self.

I've learned it's not so important to clearly define something that, as I said earlier, is beyond human comprehension. It *is* important to begin with an open mind of hope. It doesn't have to be full-blown trust yet—just hope that maybe the way I run the show without this Power or Higher Self isn't always effective.

The Big Book of Alcoholics Anonymous has a beautiful analogy to describe what happens when I'm not trusting the Mystic Law. It talks of an actor who is trying to arrange all parts of the play—the lights, the music, the other actors—in a way to suit himself. The actor is trying to play the role of director while acting.

What happens? The actor gets frustrated and tries to manipulate everything to go a certain way, which it inevitably *doesn't*. Because of this, the actor ends up exhausted and angry, while also angering and offending others around him— creating a ton of confusion and ultimately a terrible play.

When I'm able to relax and say to myself, "The Universe has my back" without gripping so tightly to controlling every outcome in my life, life runs way more smoothly, and I stop being resentful that things aren't going my way.

So I invite you now: you don't necessarily have to trust that natural flow and order, but at least suspend the belief that trusting a Higher Power or the Higher Mind or your Higher Self *won't* work. You can get to trusting this source later. Right now, I just want to inspire you to have even the tiniest bit of *hope* that there might be forces beyond you that support you in living your best life and recovering from a seemingly hopeless state of being. It worked for me, and I believe it can work for you as well.

Trust Your Instincts

It was 1999, and I was a junior in college at Rutgers. The first two years had been relatively calm. Yes, it took some time to navigate being a person with a mental illness and a college student at the same time. I wanted desperately to be a "normal" college student, so I experimented with drinking while on my medication (which never ended well). I decided to be honest with people about my diagnosis. Some ran completely in the other direction, but many supported me and stayed in my life anyway.

I was living in a set of dorms reserved for juniors and seniors. Unfortunately, I had a conflict with one of my roommates because I'd made out with a guy that she really liked, and she and the other roommates decided to kick me out. I scrambled quickly to find another roommate. Alicia, a sorority sister, told me that someone was moving out of their apartment, so I moved in.

One day I was walking down our hallway when Alicia saw someone that she knew. I looked up and saw a guy standing there with a girl. The guy had brown hair and light eyes. He was muscular in build and about six feet two. The girl facing the guy had long, thick, straight, chestnut hair. My heart started to beat faster, and I thought, "Now I'm going to have a crush on a guy who is dating someone else. Not good."

Alicia introduced me to the guy: "Emily, this is my friend George," she said. George smiled, revealing a very white set of teeth. His face reminded me a bit of the actor Joshua Jackson.

"Hey," George said warmly and waved, "and this is my friend Kate."

"Friend," I thought. "Phew." Since I now assumed that George was fair game, I quickly thought on my feet. "Hey, George, Alicia and I are redecorating a little, and we could use some help with the heavy furniture."

"Sure," George said, "I have some time now." He left Kate and came with Alicia and me into the apartment. My heart was still racing, and my palms were a bit sweaty. George was strong, and I was impressed with his biceps as he lifted one of the dressers. I was newly single and not ready to get into a new relationship, but I could tell that George would be a good friend. He left, but not before saying, "Can I have your number? We should hang out sometime."

Weeks went by, and I threw myself into my schoolwork and extracurricular activities. I was really loving the sorority and being a White Shirt, which meant I was part of the group that ran Rutgers' freshman orientation program. It was quite an honor to be a part of both groups.

A few weeks later, I was at a football game when I saw George with a group of his guy friends. I walked up to him, trying to stroll like a runway model, and I saw him staring back. "Be cool, Em," I thought.

I then reminded myself that I could only be friends with George, because I was just out of a relationship. For some reason, my intuition told me to steer clear of this guy completely. All of the alarms were going off in my mind, and I didn't know why.

"That's strange," I thought, but I ignored my inner wisdom and continued to walk in his direction.

"Hey," I said. George looked up from the game that he was pretending to be absorbed in. I walked in his direction.

"Hey," George said, and then blurted out bluntly, "I don't like the color of your shirt."

"What?" I said, surprised.

"Yeah," he continued. "It's way too red for your skin tone."

"Ok, Louis Vuitton," I quipped back at him, "thanks for the feedback." I turned on my heel and was about to walk away. "This isn't good. I'm so turned on," I thought.

"Hey," George shouted after me, "we should really hang out sometime soon. Are you around tonight?"

"I'll let you know later," I said still not fully forgiving him for the shirt comment.

Later came, and I got a call from George. "My roommates and I are watching TV in our apartment. You should really come by."

I debated this a bit. I couldn't let myself get too close to this guy. I knew he was trouble, but this made me want to run downstairs to his apartment as quickly as possible. So I did.

Men were quite confusing to me at this age, so I tended to give a lot of mixed signals. This night was no exception. As soon as I got downstairs, I sat very close to George on the couch.

"Hey," I said, placing my head on his shoulder. "What's up?"

As George leaned his body closer to mine, a tug-of-war began in my mind. I knew it was not the right thing to date George. He was blunt, rude, and totally not my type, but I could only think of how turned on I was in his presence.

"Do you wanna get out of here and hang out in my apartment upstairs?" I said, hearing the proverbial angel on my shoulder urge me to run away from this man as fast as I could.

"Sure," he said.

I grabbed his hand, and we went up to my place, where no one was home. We sat down on one of the navy blue couches in my living room, but this time I sat right on his lap.

"George," I said, "I have to tell you something, and I hope you won't judge me for it. Actually, I have to tell you two things."

"Sure," he said.

"Well, the first is that every time I become friends with a guy, for some reason they want to be more than friends, and we end up hooking up, and everything goes downhill. So I hope that we can be *just* friends."

He looked at me surprised. I was still on his lap, and I could feel his heart racing. Mine was racing too. He moved over, and I fell off of his lap and on to the couch.

"What's the other thing?" he said.

"Whaa . . . oh, yeah, right. The other thing," I said, snapping out of my momentary daze.

"Well," I said, "I'm bipolar, and I've had to be hospitalized a few times, but I'm stable now, and I'm grateful." The words came out quickly and in a very matter-of-fact way.

George looked at me taking it all in. "OK, so we'll be friends. I'm sorry you went through all of that, and I'm here for you."

I could tell something about George: he wasn't judging me. I felt my whole body start to relax.

"Yeah—friends," I said, feeling a combination of control and disappointment at the same time. I pulled up the turquoise tube top that I was wearing and got up. "I've gotta get changed and go to the gym. Thanks for understanding."

George got up and looked at me in a way that I could not interpret. "Sure," he said coolly and left the apartment, letting the door slam a bit on the way out.

A few days later, I was sitting on the couch again. It was evening, and most of my friends were out at the bar, but I was twenty, so I couldn't go yet. It was probably 10 p.m. when I heard a knock on my door. I looked through the peephole, and my heart skipped a beat. It was George. I was sitting in my pj's, but I decided to let him in. I put my hand on the silver handle of the door and took a deep breath.

I opened the door, and I could smell alcohol on his breath from a foot away. He was definitely drunk. The fact that I could not see the dysfunction of this relationship from the beginning is baffling. But I could smell something more than alcohol on his breath. It was fear that mirrored my own.

"Hey George—what's up?" I said, opening up the door to let him in. But he didn't walk in. He remained right there in the doorway.

"Em," he said, "I don't know why I'm here. I promised myself that I wouldn't come by after the bar. But I just couldn't stay there. I had to come see you. I would kiss you right now, but I know that you said that all of your guy friends have wanted a relationship with you, and I'm not going to be that guy."

I don't remember who moved in first at that point, but the next thing I knew, he kissed me. And it was more than just a kiss. Up to that point, I'd never understood what they meant when they said that a kiss could feel like fireworks on the fourth of July—but that all changed the moment he kissed me. He led me to the couch, and he kissed me some more. It was electric. The taste of alcohol on his breath, the passion—it was all absorbing. I had never been kissed like that before.

We paused for a moment, and I made my hands into a fist and opened it up while making the noise of a firework. He didn't seem to get it, so I said, "Fireworks."

He smiled, "Yeah, I know."

We continued to make out on the couch, and he carried me to my bed, still kissing me. I had never experienced anything like this before. We were both so afraid, yet so entranced by the moment. Still, I pulled back before anything too monumental could happen.

"Let's take things slow," I said.

"Yeah," he said, "I know you are right." He gave me another peck, and left my room.

I giggled, "Wait, where are you going?" I said.

"I'm taking things slow," he said.

"I know, but you forgot to say goodnight," I said.

"Oh, yeah," he said, kissing me on the forehead. "Night, Em." With that, he left.

After that night, George became a regular guest in my apartment. I had roommates, so there wasn't much privacy, so we didn't have sex. But without fail every night, he would tuck me into bed. It became our little routine. We also were spending more time during the day together as well. Still, we were "just friends" in my book, and I insisted on making sure that he knew this while still making out with him every chance I got. It must have been incredibly confusing for him.

I was confused too. Something in me was still screaming to run from him as fast as I could. I couldn't put it all together, and I was so attracted to him that I just couldn't stay away. So I didn't. I was relying upon summer to give us distance, as we both were going to our respective parents' houses for the break.

May came, and it was time to leave. I was the last to leave the apartment. I had packed up everything when George came by. "I just wanted to say goodbye," he said.

I didn't say a word. I just leaned in and kissed him passionately. We said our goodbyes. I decided I'd never see him again. That was totally it for me. "Yeah," I whispered to myself, "totally it."

The next key to becoming your Higher Self is to trust your instincts. I believe that we all have intuition. It may manifest within us in different ways, but it's there. For me, I feel things in my throat and in my gut. It's as if a big snake sits coiled in my stomach and jumps up through my intestines and my esophagus into my throat, where it bites me so hard that it stings. That's when I know that I must get quiet and listen. And today I listen hard.

When I was first getting to know George, I felt that snake. I felt the sting; I heard not just warning bells but sirens. It's something that I cannot really put into words. I just knew that I should run in the other direction, and quickly.

Yet sometimes the pull of our own inner darkness is so strong that we cannot listen to our instincts. That is the way it was with George. In Buddhism, we call these negative forces *fundamental darkness*. Fundamental darkness means that a person is unaware that they are the Buddha or that they have God within them. Nor do they believe that others have the Buddha within them as well.

I believe that all traditions have fundamental darkness. Many call it the devil. It's that force of evil that we can all tap into—the part of us that denies our own value and the value of others. It's at play in every tragedy that humans have created throughout history: shootings, assassinations, racism, war. All of that evil begins because of fundamental darkness.

During the time when I met George, I was having a good period with my mental health, but inside, I still felt I was damaged goods. I felt that because I had a mental illness, I wasn't worthy of the same kind of love that others deserved. This thought alone was quite dangerous. Ultimately it could have destroyed me. But I was and am a fighter.

How do you learn to trust your own intuition? Before acting, you need to learn to pause, get quiet, and listen. I get quiet through chanting or saying a mantra over and over again.

The mantra that I say is *nam myoho renge kyo*. It's Japanese, and I will go more into its meaning later. Every time I say *nam myoho renge kyo*, my mind becomes still enough that I can hear my own inner voice.

You don't have to use this method. Some people become quiet through other types of meditation. Some get quiet through being outdoors in nature. You need to experiment with methods of your own.

Once you do, you will have a calm, still voice come over you. This is not the same voice that you feel when you are red-hot. It's not a voice that comes from a place of emotion (regardless of what that emotion is): it comes from your deepest inner wisdom.

Learning to trust this voice is the beginning of becoming your authentic Higher Self. I invite you to try it. The next time you have a decision to make, become still. Let your mind and all of the thoughts whirling around it calm down. Let your emotions settle. Be patient with this part: it can sometimes take days or weeks. But once it happens, trust that wise voice within. If you follow this intuitive sense, I assure you, you will get on the path towards the life that you were meant to live.

Let It Be

That summer was awful for me. I was suicidal and hospitalized at Gracie Square hospital, a private hospital in New York City. It was supposed to be a great hospital, but it was horrendous. There were the powder blue walls and the pacing patients that I had come to detest.

Mom and Dad and a few college friends came to visit, but nothing was shaking me out of my depression. Mom told me that my phone was ringing a lot and that it was George leaving messages. I couldn't deal. I wanted to be loved and left alone at the same time.

Finally I decided to call him from the pay phone in the hospital. I dialed his number, and my heart was beating so fast I thought it would hop out of my chest and onto the floor. "Hi," I said in a weak voice. "It's Emily."

"Hey, what's wrong?" George said, trying to read the tone in my voice.

"I'm in the hospital for my bipolar disorder in New York City." I was so ashamed. I felt I had failed by needing the hospital again; I felt I was weak and not able to keep my life together.

"Can I visit?" he said.

"No!" I said, practically yelling. "I'll call you when I get out."

"OK," he said with a sad tone "Bye, Em."

"Bye, George," I said mirroring his tone.

I finally got home from the hospital just in time to move to my new apartment. It was in an off-campus house. Everything about that place depressed me. It was dark, cold, and dirty, even after we had someone come in to clean it.

I was living with three other girls. Mom wanted me to feel comfortable so badly that she helped me make my room beautiful. It was decorated in pale yellow with lime green accents. Large yellow balloon valences hung from each window. Mom and her friend Marcia were helping me paint the room when a knock came on the door.

I went downstairs to answer it. It was flowers from George. I rolled my eyes as I told Mom and Marcia about him. "That's so sweet that he sent flowers," Marcia said.

"No, it's not," I replied. "He's so annoying and won't leave me alone!"

Marcia and Mom just laughed. The "yellow room," as it became known later, was an indoor porch that had been converted to a bedroom. It had windows on three sides, and on the fourth side were French doors.

I was still deep in depression. It was worse than ever, and I became agoraphobic. But I did not want to stay there and drove home. George was calling a lot. I answered maybe one of every four calls.

Mom and Dad wanted me to go back to school and stay there. They wanted me to finish my college education.

"Why don't you go back up to school and hang out with George? He seems to really miss you," Mom said.

I agreed to go. I called George and asked him to meet me by my apartment, where he became a regular visitor. I wasn't going out on my own, so George would come by to motivate me. He'd take me food shopping or to run errands. He was becoming my best friend.

One day, we were both cuddling on my bed. "Em," he said, "I love you. I don't want to be your friend. I need to be more. If you won't be my girlfriend, I need to get out of your life and stop being friends with you." With that, he got up and left.

I began to cry hysterically. I didn't know what to do. On the one hand, I loved George and was attracted to him. But I was so sick, and I didn't trust myself to make a good choice in that state. I also still had this nagging feeling that he was not the right person for me and that it might be good to get him out of my life. Yet I had grown dependent on him.

Coinciding with all of this, during this time my parents were advised by therapists to take a tough line with me. I wasn't allowed to come home from school, because every time I went home, I regressed and begged my parents to let me drop out of school and come home. They were against this and did everything in their power to get me to stay, including this new rule about not coming home.

"They don't love you," George said one day, referring to my parents. "I do. If they did love you, they would be here like I am.

Your friends have disappeared too," he said. "I'm the only one that loves you and wants to be here for you. Don't forget that."

I felt so rejected by my family, and so helpless, and there was George, taking care of me. I couldn't lose him. He loved me in a way that I had never been loved before.

"OK, George," I said soon after this conversation, "I'll be your girlfriend."

He didn't say a thing but kissed me passionately.

"Em," he said after a while, "there is something else. I really am worried about you. I know that if you don't convert from Judaism to my religion, you will go to hell. I really need to save you from this!"

"What?" I said, shocked. "I'm not doing that!"

"But Em," he said, "you said that you barely practiced Judaism."

"I know," I said, "but I'm not converting. I'm Jewish, and will always be."

"Well, then I can't introduce you to my family. You are too sick, and you are living in hell. I won't introduce you to them until you let me save you."

"George, that's so unfair," I said. "How can you call me your girlfriend but not want to introduce me to your parents?"

But he wouldn't budge on this.

"OK," I said coolly, "then I won't be your girlfriend."

And with that, I rolled over and looked the other way.

"Fine!" he said, getting dressed quickly, and stormed out slamming the French doors.

This lasted for almost two days. I was so depressed that I didn't shower and didn't leave the yellow room for anything but food.

"George," I said finally over the phone, "I'm just upset because I want to marry you, and I won't know that you are serious about marrying me until you introduce me to your parents."

"Em," George said laughing, "you're not even twenty-one years old yet. I'm going to marry you, but we have a lot of time for that."

"OK," I said. "Let's get back together."

"OK," he said, "I'm coming right over."

Even with George to "love" me, I was struggling immensely. I had dropped out of all but one class. I was still experiencing suicidal depression, and I was in and out of the hospital like a revolving door. I tried working at a local hair salon, and my condition improved slightly, but I was still struggling. Then I was fired from that job, and off into the hospital I went.

This cycle kept repeating itself, and so did my cycle of breaking up and getting back together with George. The more intense the relationship got, the more I tried to run away, and the more George tried to cling to me.

"George," I would say, "Please! They say if you love something, let it go, and if it's meant to be, it will come back to you."

"Em," George said, "that's bullshit. I believe if you love someone, cling to them as tightly as possible."

Don't get me wrong: it wasn't always fighting and difficulty between us. We had some great times; some of the highest points of my life—the best days—were by his side. Yet there were the fights.

"Em," he'd say, screaming at me, "You are evil, evil, evil."

"George," I would cry, "why do you think that?"

"Because, Em, you are putting me through hell, and you keep on breaking up with me."

It was so confusing. The more I got well, the more intense the screaming got. But it would be sandwiched in by moments so sublime and lovely that I just couldn't leave him. Still, I felt that he didn't trust me completely. He stuck hard to the line drawn in the sand that he wouldn't introduce me to his parents unless I truly got well from my mental illness and converted.

The year went by, and I spent my summer studying abroad without him, which felt quite liberating. For that whole summer, I was not symptomatic at all. Yet as soon as I returned back from that trip, I was back in the hospital again. I couldn't stay stable, no matter how badly I wanted it.

I also wasn't sleeping. I would stay at George's a couple of nights out of the week, and I just could never fall asleep there. My mind would race. Should I be with George, or should I bolt? Why doesn't he want me to be a part of his family life? And why does he yell at me so much?

One day we were in the middle of a big fight, and George left the room to get ready for bed. He couldn't get his contacts out, and got so angry that he pulled the sink out of the bathroom wall. It was a really bad moment, not just for him, but for me. But still I loved him.

It was probably my eighth hospitalization at this point. George did cling to me and stayed at my side through all of it.

The hospitalization was particularly rough this time. The doctors took me off my benzodiazepine medication, which reduced my anxiety and helped me sleep, because it was addictive. I had had so many hospitalizations that they were threatening to lock me away in the state hospital. I was so sick that the other patients on the floor called me "crazy" to my face.

I stopped eating. George loyally came to visit me. There must have been so much pressure on him. He was young and was trying to finish his senior year of college and get a job. I would go into the hospital, and everyone would tell me to leave him for good. Then he'd beg to visit, and I would finally break down. This cycle played out over and over, and this hospitalization was no exception.

I remember him walking onto the floor. He looked great. He was wearing a black J. Crew sweater and jeans that showed off his butt. I was powerfully attracted to him. As he walked in, one of the other girls said, "Is that your man? You should hold onto that one and don't let go."

I went up to him and kissed and hugged him. I loved the way he hugged. It was going to be different from this point forward; I just knew it.

He walked past one of the patients who had been court-ordered to be there, named John. John was a hippie and weighed probably over 300 pounds. He was always asking people to get him out of there.

"He's cool," George said as he walked by, and I knew he meant it. George was very open-minded in that way.

He came into my room and kissed me. "Em, I miss you so much," he said sweetly.

"I know," I said, "I miss you too. If I ever get out of here, it will be awesome to come back to you. But I really want to talk about this marriage thing. Why won't you introduce—" but before I could get out more, he put his fingers to my lips.

"Em," he said, "relax, relax. Don't get yourself all upset now. You need to heal."

An acoustic guitar could be heard in the distance at that moment. Someone was singing "Let It Be" by the Beatles.

"Em," George said, "let's just let it be for now," and with that he took my hand and lead me towards the music. It turned out that John had a friend who had come to visit with his acoustic guitar and was leading a sing-along. George sat down, and I sat on his lap.

We began singing, and George swayed back and forth, with me still on his lap. I felt a warmth that I hadn't felt in a long time. Not with George, not with anyone. I was alive again. And I knew I loved and was loving in return. That was all that mattered for now.

The next key to becoming your best self is to know when to let it be. One of the main themes that ran through my life was trying to control everything around me. I had no faith whatsoever, so I believed that in order to make things work out, I had to *make* them work.

I decided that I wanted to marry George right after college. After all, that's how it worked out for my parents. I obsessed about this so hard that I couldn't see the problems right in front of my face. I knew that George and I were dysfunctional, but I assumed that this would fix itself as we continued to work on the relationship.

In the end, obsessing about marrying George and trying to force it just didn't work. I had to learn that I couldn't control the Universe. I had to learn that there were higher forces in operation. I had to learn how to slow down and let things flow. But during the worst parts of my mental illness, I had no capacity to do this.

I invite you to take a good look at your life right now. Do you need to let go of certain things and turn them over to the Universe? Are there areas where you are not trusting? Are there areas where you are fighting so hard for something but keep coming up against closed doors?

There is a reason for this. The Higher Mind knows more than you know about the way things are meant to work out. We can see only a sliver of the possibilities available to us. We think that we know what we need, but many times we have no idea what will truly make us happy and will be the best outcome for the world.

Once one of my favorite songs was by the Rolling Stones: "You Can't Always Get What You Want." The song talks about how you don't always get what you want in life, but if you really think about it, "you get what you need."

I used to hate it when George reminded me of this song, but he was right. The human mind is not capable of seeing all the different ways their life can go. When we learn to trust the Universe, that's when things start to really flow. It takes too much energy to plot, plan, and scheme. When we "let go and let God," as they say in the Twelve Step programs, the results are much better, and we don't grow so tired out by life. In fact, we *get* energy from going with the flow of life. From that energy, amazing things can happen. We can be more present for our spouses. We can be more grateful for the here and now and all the abundance that we have in our lives for the moment. We can rest easy, knowing that we don't have to be in charge at all times. Most importantly, when we connect to our Source in this way, we can hear what is most authentic about ourselves and be present for the nudges that the Universe gives us to direct us towards our highest purpose.

The end of "Let It Be" promises us that "there will be an answer." But this answer doesn't come from racking our brains and trying to think our way through a problem. It comes from getting quiet, letting go of trying to fix things right away, and allowing them to work out for themselves.

I'm not advocating inaction. I'm saying that we want to listen to the Universe and connect our hearts and minds to it. That is when the answers come.

Key 7

Find Your Mentors

It's three o'clock in the afternoon, and I've just been released from the hospital. It's 2001, and I am twenty-two years old and a senior in college. The hospitalization has been particularly rough this time. I came out of it a broken woman.

I'm now waiting in the waiting room of the outpatient center at Rutgers New Jersey Medical School's University Behavioral Health clinic. The center has a cold feel to it. The walls are tan cinderblock, and there are prints of artists like Monet thrown hastily up on the walls. The receptionists are sitting unresponsively behind thick glass.

Today is the day that I'll meet my new outpatient therapist. It's an important day, because I cannot stand the thought of going back into the hospital again, and I know I need help to learn how to stay out of it. As much as I hate the hospital, I feel I have no other place to turn when I have suicidal thoughts and want to act on them. I have no idea how I'm going to avoid this hospital, but I know it needs to happen so that I don't end up in the state hospital.

People who have been in the state hospital have described it to me. If the hospitals I've been in are hell, the state hospital sounds like being in jail in hell. You must watch your back at all times. No activities, terrible food, and no end date to your release. I don't want my life to end up this way. It seems like a total waste of an existence.

Not knowing what else to do, I begin to pray. "God," I say in my head, "if you exist, please let this therapist help me to change my situation. Please help me to help myself."

I finish, and the receptionist calls my name.

"Emily Grossman," she says brusquely, "room four."

I get up timidly and walk to room four. I'm a hollow shell lying helplessly on the bottom of an ocean of sadness. I walk into the room, and there is Meghna.

"Hello," she says meekly. "My name is Meghna, and I'll be your new therapist."

I immediately start crying in sheets of tears. "My life is falling apart, and I don't know what to do," I sob. "They've already said that if I go into the hospital again, they will send me to the state hospital."

Meghna becomes visibly panicked by my sobbing. She reaches for her phone. I know what's coming. She's going to send me right back into the hospital. Before she can dial, I run out of the room and speak to the receptionist through the hole in the bottom of the glass.

"This isn't going to work," I say, cursing God for not answering my prayers. "She can't help me. I'm not going to leave this clinic until you get me another therapist, and a good one!" I say in my strongest voice. I don't know what gives me the fortitude to advocate so heavily for myself, but I don't have the time to question it.

The receptionist looks stunned and picks up her phone immediately.

"Shit," I think, "that's it for me. Off to the state hospital I go."

The receptionist, trying to remain professional, hangs up the phone. "OK, go back into room four, Miss Grossman," she says in an unemotional tone.

Surprised and confused, I skulk back to the room. Meghna is still sitting there, and I'm majorly disappointed.

"Well, that didn't work," I think.

As if she is reading my mind, Meghna says, "My supervisor is coming in a moment."

Just as she says this, the door flies open, letting in bright light, and in walks a very stylish and professional-looking woman in her early fifties. She has straight black hair cut into a perfect bob. She is wearing edgy red glasses and a black dress with high black leather boots. She sits down, and already I can sense in her energy that she is a force of nature.

"I'm Sherrie Schwab. What is the problem here?" she asks in a businesslike tone.

I'm still sobbing, and trying to answer her through my tears.

"Oh, no!" she says sternly, pointing at me with her red, manicured index finger. "You are a grown woman. You sit up, stop crying, and tell me like an adult what is wrong."

She holds out a tissue box, and I grab a tissue and do my best to suck back my sobs. "I just got out of the hospital, and I feel like I'm broken, and I'm afraid to go to the state hospital, and I hate myself and my life," I say, and start sobbing again.

"OK," she says. "I am a very busy woman, but I have one time slot available for you to take, under one condition: that you act like the young woman that you are. All this crying is what kids do. You are an adult, and you are not sick! I'll see you next Wednesday at 3 p.m."

And with that, she hands me her card, turns on her heel, and leaves the room. I don't even question it. I don't look at my schedule. I just know that whatever it takes, I *must* be there at 3 p.m. the following Wednesday. God has answered me and brought in the big guns, and I know that I have no choice but to listen.

After what seems like eons, Wednesday at 3 p.m. finally comes. I walk into Sherrie's office, but I'm five minutes late.

"Emily," she says peering at me through her red glasses, "being late is therapy-interfering behavior."

I don't know why I don't snap back, which is my usual tendency when confronted, but I don't. Instead, I look into Sherrie's dark eyes, which are looking at me through those red glasses like those of a wise owl.

"I'm sorry."

"Now," she says, "it says from your hospital record that you have borderline personality disorder. Do you know what that is?"

I nod, ashamed. Borderline personality disorder is a diagnosis describing labile moods, difficulty connecting with others, and a ton of suicidal thoughts and threats to act on them. I don't agree that this is my diagnosis. I hate everything about it; the name makes it sound as if I'm about to jump off the edge of something, but not before I bring everyone else with me. I think about a movie in which Glenn Close plays a character with this diagnosis, and she boils her boyfriend's bunny. I want nothing to do with it.

"Here's the good news," Sherrie says matter-of-factly. "This qualifies you not only to see me weekly but to attend a group that I am running called dialectical behavior therapy. Ever heard of it?"

"No," I say. I hate groups: they are a lot of complaining with no solutions. Yet something about Sherrie makes me listen. It's not just her tone; it's her presence. I feel totally safe, yet challenged much in the way I felt in the presence of Mrs. Collins all those years ago. I don't know how, but I recognize Sherrie as my new mentor—the person who will bring me out of the hell that I've been living in for far too long. For the first time in a long time, I have hope.

There is an old saying: "When the student is ready, the teacher appears." This is exactly how I feel about this next key to becoming one's best self. At every turn at which I became ready to develop an aspect of myself, the perfect mentor has appeared to guide me through it. I have been blessed with some profound mentors. Mrs. Collins was a mentor for my writing. When I was ready for a mentor around my mental health, in walked Sherrie Schwab. I could go on.

What makes a good mentor? The most important thing is that there must be a soul connection. You almost feel as if you were together before (and in my opinion, you probably have been, in other lifetimes). Often, time seems to stop when you first meet them, and later you can remember your first meeting quite vividly.

Besides this soul connection—this feeling that you've known the person before and the ease with which you both communicate—there also usually is a purpose for being together that you figure out relatively quickly. It's not a relationship where two equals are coming together to create something new. It's more of a teacher-student relationship, where one person clearly has something to teach the other. Many other relationships can feel like soul connections, but in this kind, the mentor is there to teach something to the mentee. Nevertheless, it's an even exchange of energy in that the mentor gets as much from the experience as the mentee, just by watching the mentee progress.

You may think you value independence above all else and don't need to be taught things; you'll just figure them out on your own. It's true that you can, but I guarantee that having a mentor is a great shortcut. It's also part of the universal flow of things. Look in nature. A bird needs to be fed and encouraged to fly by its mother. Flowers are pollinated by bees. Squirrels spread acorns, which turn into trees. Humans too require support at various junctures in their growth if they are truly trying to become their best selves.

I do not advise anyone to have merely one mentor. Life is multifaceted, and no one person has the answers to everything. To rely on one person alone takes us away from our connection to the Universe. Yet it's valuable to find people to support you in areas that are important to your growth.

A mentor doesn't even have to be someone you know. It can be someone whose values you respect and on whom you can model your life. Many of my friends have said that even though they don't know Oprah Winfrey, she has been their mentor. They have become better people because they live their lives as she has, with her grace, compassion, and love for others. I am not here to tell you who your mentor should be. It's a deeply personal choice. But I am suggesting that you find someone you admire and can grow with. Growth is an essential part of becoming your best self, and a mentor can show you how.

⊶━━ Key 8

Move Forward No Matter What

September 11, 2001. I was a senior in college, and still twenty-two, when the world changed forever. Two planes crashed into the Twin Towers in New York City. The effect was felt throughout the world, but those of us who were living so close felt it very deeply.

I remember that day well. I was back in college, taking a full-time course load. I was just four courses away from graduation. George and I were still dating, although things had gone from bad to worse. He had moved home and gotten his first job. The distance shouldn't have meant as much as it did, but he was very worried that I would meet another man while he was away. He was angrier than ever. Although I was deeply in love with him, I didn't know how to handle his rage. The yelling just wouldn't stop. I'd be on the phone with him late into the evening, and my roommates would look at me in disbelief.

"I can hear him screaming at you over the phone," one of them said. "Why don't you just leave him?"

"I love him," I said, and went storming out of the room.

Anyway, 9/11 was a horrible day for all. My father and sister Pam were in New York City, and I wasn't sure if I'd ever see them again. Pam got off the train in New Jersey first. She and mom came right up to school and sat in my room. We were waiting to hear from Dad. Classes were canceled. The air was heavy.

I called George. Because of his proximity to New York City, one could hear sirens everywhere. It was all hands on deck. "Can you come here?" I said, crying.

"No, Em," he said in hysterics. "I have to be here for my family."

George and his family were shaken by the events. I tried to understand, but deep inside I couldn't have felt more separate from George during this crisis. I had met his mother the year before, during his graduation, but she still only thought of me as his friend. We were living separate lives.

This is when the psychosis began. Psychosis can manifest in many different ways. In my case, I became delusional in my thinking and was seeing and hearing things that weren't there. My delusions began to center around 9/11.

Homecoming came, and I didn't go. I had been having trouble doing basic things, even cooking for myself. I had some chicken one night, and my delusions told me that I was poisoned by anthrax, which at that time was thought to be sent through the mail as a form of terrorism. I began going from door to door in my New Brunswick, New Jersey, neighborhood ringing bells to try and find an antidote.

Finally, a man answered the door. He was dressed in a chef's outfit.

"Hi," I said to this total stranger. "Can I come in? I think I'm poisoned by anthrax."

The guy laughed, "Sure. C'mon in," he said in a friendly tone. While the details of what happened next are a bit hazy, I will do my best to relay what I remember.

"What's your name?" the guy said.

"I'm Emily," I said.

"Well, Emily, I don't think you have anthrax poisoning. I think you have food poisoning. Here, why don't you take this?" he said, handing me a square tablet.

"Ok," I said, desperate for what I now know were delusions to stop. I'll never know what the guy really gave me, but I suspect it was an acid tab.

"Why don't you lay down on my bed and rest a little bit until this passes?" the guy said, and I obliged.

I'm not sure if I slept, or what happened next, but soon the guy was standing over me and looking at me. Except in my mind, it wasn't him; it was my ex-boyfriend from high school.

"Jay?" I cried, so relieved to see him. But before I could give him a hug, the face changed again. Now it was one of my male elementary school friends.

I got up, put on my shoes, and ran out of the house screaming.

"Emily!" the man called after me. But it was too late. Outside there were police officers waiting. I tried to outrun them, and I was in very good shape, but in this trippy delusional state, I didn't get far. I was trapped like a rat almost instantly.

Two of the male police officers grabbed me. I tried to struggle, but it was no use. They were bigger and stronger than me.

One of the officers laughed as he pulled out a straitjacket. "Looks like we've got a live one here, Mark."

Mark and the other officer chuckled as they stuffed my arms into the stiff sleeves of the straitjacket and buckled each buckle. They then pushed me into the back seat of the police car, still joking with each other about me.

"I'm so glad I'm a source of entertainment for these assholes," I thought in a lucid moment.

They brought me into the ER screaming and howling. I was screaming for George, I was screaming for my parents, I was screaming for anyone who could get me out of yet another hospitalization. Then I felt a strong prick, and I knew what they had done: they had shot me up with a tranquilizer.

The next thing I remember was being on a hard bed with metal all around it in an isolated room. I prayed at this moment, harder than I had ever prayed. "Please, God, if you can bring me to, and get me out of this mess, I promise to be loyal to you forever."

It seemed to work. I was there on that hard bed overnight. I felt numb and drowsy from whatever tranquilizer they gave me.

I remembered what Sherrie Schwab had told me: "Emily, you are not sick. You don't need the hospital." I believed her.

It was time to be questioned by hospital admissions. This was the make it or break it moment: what I said to this woman would determine if I was able to go home and continue with my classes towards graduation or not. I was determined to graduate no matter what. I stood up ready to do battle.

I entered a dark room with wood paneling on the walls. It was an ugly, cold room, and seated in the center of it was Mrs. Wilson, who was the gatekeeper in the admissions department of the hospital.

"Hello, I'm Mrs. Wilson," the woman said strictly. "Have a seat."

"Ms. Grossman," she said, "do you know where you are and what time it is?"

Groan. I hated this routine, which I knew so well. First, they need to see if you are oriented in time and place. Luckily, I had looked at the clock in the isolation room ahead of time.

"Yeah. I'm at University Behavioral Health Center in Piscataway, New Jersey. It's 10 a.m.," I said defiantly.

"Ms. Grossman, that's fine, but I'd like you to check the attitude," Mrs. Wilson said. Going on, she said, "Where are you from, and where do you live now?"

"I'm from Marlboro, New Jersey and I live in New Brunswick, New Jersey. I'm a student at Rutgers College," I said.

"Hmmm," she said, "I used to live in Marlboro, New Jersey. I hung out at the convenience store right there on Route 79 with my friends all the time."

I knew she was bluffing. They often used this technique to see if you were too vulnerable and out of touch with reality to be released. There was no way that this woman was from Marlboro. I could smell the arrogance and affluence of Marlboro from a mile away, and this woman didn't have it.

"You're not from Marlboro," I said calling Mrs. Wilson on her bullshit.

"Yeah, yeah, I am, man. I loved it by them horse farms," Mrs. Wilson insisted.

By this point, I was annoyed. "Fine," I said, "if you are from Marlboro, what was the mascot of Marlboro High School?" I asked, undeterred.

Mrs. Wilson laughed so hard she snorted. "Very clever," she said. "Any thoughts of hurting yourself or others?" she continued.

"Nope," I said. I knew that I had already triumphed.

"Ok, Ms. Grossman," Mrs. Wilson said. "I'll call you a cab. You are free to go."

I sighed, extremely relieved. I had no time for another hospitalization. I had to graduate, and fast. I was already a year and a half behind schedule, and I couldn't wait to be done with Rutgers.

As soon as I got back, I called George. "Hey, hon," I said, "you are never going to believe what just happened. It was so awful. I thought I was poisoned by anthrax, and I went into the guy's house and . . ."

"What?" George said interrupting me, "you were in some random guy's house? Were you cheating on me?" By this point he was screaming.

"No, babe," I said, "please calm down!" but it was too late.

"Do you know how fucked up you are?" he yelled. "You go into some random guy's house and hook up with him. I can't believe you. You're the worst girlfriend in the whole world. You're the worst person in the whole world! You're pure evil. No, you're worse than evil."

"Babe," I tried to interject, "I didn't—"

"Em," George interrupted, "you're so lucky I stay with you. You're a worthless piece of shit." He was yelling louder than I had ever heard him yell before.

"I gotta go, honey," I said, crying, "I'm really nauseous."

I hung up and ran right into the bathroom, where I threw up. This had become more and more common. Every time he acted like this, my stomach got upset, and I threw up.

I brushed my teeth and came out of the bathroom. My housemates were just coming home from homecoming. "Em," one of them said, "was that George screaming at you? Why the hell do you stay with him?"

By this point I was in tears, so I pushed passed them and ran into my room. What the hell was I going to do? I had no support besides George. My parents were in and out of my life, as instructed by my therapist. My sister and all of my friends were keeping their distance. I couldn't leave George. He was the only support I had. But this was too much, and I needed to graduate.

I called George back, "Hey hon, can you please come down here when you are able to? We need to talk this out face-to-face." George agreed to come down over the weekend.

The weekend came, and it was time for George to come down. I was terrified of how things would go. But something needed to change. It just couldn't go on like this.

I pulled up to my house in my red Toyota Celica and screamed. There was George in a black leather jacket and aviator sunglasses sitting in a chair in the backyard. I was expecting him, but at this point, I was terrified of him.

"Hey," he said, trying to kiss me as I got out of the car. But I pulled away. "What the hell, Em!" he shouted as we went inside.

"Babe, please keep your voice down. You're going to bother my roommates! C'mon, let's go into my room."

We sat on my bed. "I just can't do it anymore," I said, crying. George started crying too. Somehow this was different from the other times I had broken up with him. We were both tired, I think.

"Em," he said through tears, "I feel like we're going back to the beginning when I was chasing after you. I can't keep doing this."

"So don't," I said, "We need to break up. I need to graduate, and you need to move on."

I didn't want this, but I knew I wouldn't graduate this way. It was too distracting. George got up and headed for the door. Just as he was about to leave, I reached out to squeeze his hand. "I love you," I said.

"So fucked up," was his reply, as he pulled his hand away and slammed the screen door.

The rest of the semester was awful. I was still struggling with psychosis. My roommates didn't know what to make of it and would shout, "Jeepers, creepers," to my face every time I came into the room. I was desperate to have love and support, but everywhere I turned, people were running away, horrified by my bizarre behavior. I didn't want to admit it, but I missed George's "love" and support more than ever.

Then the week before I was supposed to graduate, my grandmother was in the hospital.

"Hello, love," Grandma Trudy said in an uncharacteristically weak voice. "Can you come to visit me?"

"Grandma," I said, crying, "I can't. I have one more week and so many papers to write! I love you, though."

That was the last time I would see my Grandma Trudy, whom I loved dearly. She died the next day.

"Sherrie," I said, crying over the phone to my therapist, "I just can't take anymore! I can't do it. This is too hard."

"Emily," Sherrie said, "please come back to the moment. I know that you are grieving a lot of things right now, but you are close to graduation. If you don't finish now, you will get so caught up with Grandma and grieving that you may never finish."

I knew that she was right. It had taken everything I had to continue school while experiencing psychosis, and I knew I needed to finish. I handed in my last paper as quickly as possible and then rushed down to West Long Branch, New Jersey, to be with my family.

The next key to becoming one's Higher Self is to keep going no matter what. During the time that I was experiencing psychosis, and many other times during my battle with mental illness, I was tempted to give up. Sometimes this would take the form of suicidal thoughts. At other times, I merely wanted to drop out of college.

Regardless, there was something within me that knew to keep on moving forward. Life can get difficult at times: it can deal blows that are unfathomable. When I was working on my final papers, experiencing psychosis, being bullied and mocked by my roommates, had just had a bad breakup, and had lost my grandmother, I would have been justified in giving up. But I wouldn't.

My family motto is, "*Nos Grossmani nunquam desperamus*," which is Latin for, "We Grossmans never give up." I have never forgotten this. During the times where life has had me up against the wall, I've learned to dig in harder.

I've heard it said that the only way out is through. I find a great deal of wisdom in this saying. Life is not about avoiding problems or working around them: that's impossible. Instead it's about learning to dive headfirst into the fire, feel you've been almost burned alive, and come out the other side, scars and all. The scars harden and become callouses that remind us of the pain while also reminding us that we are capable of getting through it. And these callouses give us our power.

I used to think that in order to overcome my mental illness, I had to take a break from life. I imagined traveling someplace different or going to a luxurious treatment center for a couple of years until I was "fully healed" and ready to continue with life.

In hindsight, I know that that would have been the worst thing for me. There's no such thing in life as "fully healed." We are never truly whole. Like a beating heart, life simply expands and contracts, giving us highs and lows throughout the journey. The key is to just persevere, no matter what. Forward motion and time are the true healers. This is living in the solution rather than dwelling on the problem. When we continue with the forward momentum, no matter what, the Universe comes in to help us to work things out.

Build and Use Your Skills

It's the summer of 2002. I'm twenty-three years old and sitting with Sherrie in her new office, having a therapy session. Sherrie has begun her own private practice. Her office is decorated in primary colors, and I'm sitting on her red leather couch. The couch is cold from the air conditioning, but I'm so sweaty from outside that the skin on my legs is stuck to it.

I'm not doing well at all. I have been in the hospital about ten times, and I'm miserable. But, I'm staying the course with Sherrie. She is smart, and she gets to the heart of what is bothering me.

Unlike other therapists, Sherrie refuses to get psychoanalytical with me. We don't dig down into my deep dark past. We simply see what is going on in my life presently and how I can overcome current obstacles. It's hard for me to stay in the present, but Sherrie is strict with me and brings me back to the present every time I drift.

While I'm not applying any of it, I've been in a dialectical behavior therapy (DBT) class with Sherrie, where I've learned a lot of strategies to manage my intense emotions and difficult interpersonal situations. The class is great. I've participated, done my homework, and taken careful notes. But using what I'd learned after class was over is a choice that I've been refusing to make.

Because of the class, I've been able to break out of my relationship with George. But I'm still mourning this loss. Relationships are so complicated.

Back in Sherrie's office, she is trying to remind me to look at the chain of events leading up to my current hysteria. She sits next to me on the couch and starts drawing something that looks like a chain. She says, "OK, Emily, write down what happened, using one link of the chain per event."

I start to do this, and I'm getting more and more upset as I'm writing. Sherrie tries to calm me down, but it's no use: I'm hysterical. Sherrie gets strict again with me. "Emily, you need to use your skills."

I look at her perplexed, not sure what she is talking about. "Emily, in each chain reaction, you can use skills to not up the ante and make things worse."

I continue to look puzzled, so Sherrie, raising her voice, explains: "Emily, if you don't want your emotions to get more and more intense, you need to use some of the coping strategies or skills that you have been learning to interrupt the chain. The sooner you use skills during a series of negative events, the sooner you can prevent your emotions from getting out of control.

"Let's look at the current link in the chain of your problem from today," Sherrie continues. "It starts when you and your mother had a disagreement. Right then you had a choice point. You could either get worked up or use a skill to calm your emotions. What skill could you have used?" she says.

"I really like the mindfulness strategies, like breathing, and coming back to the present moment," I say, finally understanding it.

"Yes!" Sherrie says. "Now let's go further. Let's say that you didn't use your skills then. The next link in the chain is that you went and got some icing at a store and started binge-eating it. Let's say that you wanted to prevent yourself from taking things further and letting your emotions get out of control then. What could you have done?"

"I could have used a distraction technique, like reading a book or writing something. Then I wouldn't have started feeling so worthless that I would have started binge eating and have suicidal thoughts again. I could also have used radical acceptance. I don't have to like that I ate the icing, but rather than beating myself up about it, I could have accepted it and moved forward."

"Exactly," Sherrie says.

I wish that I could say that right then and there I decided to use those skills always, but that's not the case. Yet I at least realized that my emotions didn't have to be in charge of me: I could be in charge of them by using skills.

Sherrie used to say, "You can ride the horse, or you can let it ride you." She meant that either you can let your emotions get out of control and control you or you can take control of them.

Later in my recovery journey, I would start using the skills more consistently. This is when the magic happened. This is when I learned to take control of my emotions and really recover from mental illness.

The next key to becoming your Higher Self is to build and use your coping skills. Both are equally important. If you don't have these skills, how can you use them? That's why you have to build and then practice them, especially when nothing really negative is going on in your life. Meditation has become one of my coping strategies. I know that I can't wait until a crisis hits to meditate; I have to do it every day, consistently. That way I'm in the habit and I've practiced enough to do it well in the crisis.

The same is true of any coping skill. If I'm not used to breathing techniques, when a crisis hits, I'm not going to use that skill successfully, because my body and mind won't be used to it. There is a comfort that comes with using a coping strategy that I've practiced a thousand times before. When I need it, my body and mind know that it's a cue to relax and let go of the buildup of emotions.

Here is a list of some of my favorite coping strategies. I'm not telling you that these are the ones that you should use, because what works for me might not work for you. But start building up an arsenal of them. This way, if one doesn't work at a particular time, you can go down the list and find another.

1. Breathing techniques.
2. Coming back to the present moment over and over.
3. Talking to my dad about the problem.

4. Talking to anyone who will validate my emotions and not tell me to get over it.
5. Writing about the problem and finding solutions through reflection.
6. Chanting.
7. Walking.
8. Dancing.
9. Weight lifting.
10. Petting my cats.
11. Remembering that I've solved problems like this before.
12. Accepting that things are as they are meant to be.
13. Seeing what I can learn from the problem.
14. Listening to a Louise Hay guided meditation on YouTube.
15. Doing a creative project.
16. Helping someone else.
17. Going to a Buddhist meeting.
18. Watching funny videos on my phone.
19. Being at a beach (in the summertime).
20. Doing my hair and getting dressed up when I feel like staying in bed (doing the opposite of what I feel like doing).

I could go on. These are my top twenty favorite skills, but I'm always looking for and adding new ones. I never want to get caught in a situation where I don't have enough skills to try when I really need them.

These skills are not just for people with mental illness. Everyone has problems and emotions, so everyone needs skills. Successful, evolved people are people who use skills to

manage their intense emotions. Think about it: if you dis-
agree with your boss and you get into a big argument with
her, you could lose your job. But, if you manage your emotions, chances are the problem will work out, and you will
keep your job. Skills are for everyone. The more adept that
you get at using them, the happier, and closer to your Higher
Self you will become.

⊶——🔑 Key 10

Use the Law of Inertia

It's early in the afternoon in the spring of 2003. I have recently graduated from Rutgers. After a failed first attempt at work, I am living in a supported housing situation, which means that I am living with other people with mental illness, and a case worker checks up on us weekly.

George and I have not gotten back together, but we are still hanging out from time to time and talking fairly regularly. It's dramatic and painful. Every time we hang out, I tell him that we can't do this anymore, and he agrees. We swear that it's the last time we are going to see each other, only to come back again for more. I want to get back together, but he does not. It's a hellish existence for me, and probably for him as well.

I do things that I'm not proud of to try to get George back, including showing up to his parent's house uninvited. My self-worth is at an all-time low, and I'm desperate for some-one to tell me that I'm lovable. This charade with George will go on for the next six or seven years before he finally cuts me off for good.

I'm looking out the dirty window in my shared apartment in Freehold, New Jersey. The place is rundown and cheap and looks as if it hasn't been redecorated in forty years. I am there because after twelve hospitalizations, I have officially become a mental patient. I have also narrowly escaped being institu-tionalized in a state hospital for life.

My roommates all have schizophrenia and can often be heard laughing or talking to themselves as they go about their days, as if responding to some internal conversation that I'm not privy to. We don't really have true days. We all sit on the ugly, rough plaid couch, maybe watching TV or staring into space, but never talking to each other. We are four strangers, and we will stay that way.

It's a Wednesday, and I'm sitting on that couch. Time goes by slowly, like molasses oozing out of the jar. Suddenly one of my roommates opens the front door and comes running in.

"Emily, you have a package," she says excitedly. She hands me a rectangular brown parcel and waits expectantly. I realize that she wants to see what it is, and I move to my room, par-tially to spite her and partially to protect my privacy.

My hands are clammy as I rip the rough brown pack-ing paper and look at the package inside. It's from my sister Pam. Man, I miss her. We were very close growing up, but as I retreated deeper and deeper into bipolar disorder, our rela-tionship became less and less deep. In fact, I am very surprised that she has sent me something.

The package turns out to be a book. As I handle the shiny green cover, I feel the chills come over me. *Awaken the Giant Within* is the title, and it's by a self-help guru named Tony Robbins. My attention span is shot (a symptom of my illness), but I start to read the intro and become acquainted with this man. While the details of this book are now hazy, my spirit senses something: Tony Robbins is one of those people that are often known as "wounded healers." He has come from a time when he had no job, no close relationships, and no real life and has become the Tony Robbins that the world knows today: confident, successful, and helpful to the world.

A light bulb goes off for me, and I think, "Why not me?" This may seem like a grandiose thought, and it is, but it's not one that leads to my usual delusional thinking. It's something else—a thought that leads to action.

What is to follow is not a miraculous turnaround of the sort you would see in a movie montage, where the mental patient instantly becomes transformed into a female Tony Robbins. Even so, a spark of hope comes over me and arouses feelings that have been dead for a long time: feelings of life, possibility, and hope.

Tony Robbins' intro (I confess that I didn't get much beyond that part of the book) puts me back in motion. It won't solve everything for me, but it inspires me to start to try again.

Another key, which I learned in high-school physics, is inertia. For an object at rest to start moving, there needs to be an outside push, called an impetus. The law of inertia also says that an object in motion stays in motion. The intro to *Awaken the Giant Within* was my impetus.

Another key to moving towards your Higher Self is taking action. If you are feeling stuck right now, the best thing you can do is think of the first baby step towards your dreams and take it. Break your dream life into its most essential ingredients, and then break that down even more. Then think of a small first action step.

I will illustrate how this works. When I was living in the shared apartment in Freehold, became inspired by Tony Robbins, and had the thought, "Why not me?" it was just that: a thought. Yes, it was a positive thought, and the first one that I'd had in a while. But thoughts have little power if they are not acted upon. Had I not taken a small baby step after that, the thought would have been drowned out right away by a million other negative and defeatist thoughts, and I would have stayed stuck on that old plaid couch.

Instead, the first thing that I did was run to my closet. I knew I had a suit from my college years, and I tried it on to see if it still fit, which it did. I looked at myself in the mirror and visualized myself on a job interview. This was baby step number one.

It was a very subtle step, but it got me in motion. It broke into all of the negativity and doubt and moved me just an inch. Yet it really wasn't just an inch. This action had created a leap from hopelessness to the land of possibility. With that one action, I had crossed the gap between being a mental patient for life and moving myself towards success.

I didn't know this at the time, but I felt this subtle shift. It was as if by suiting up, I was saying to the Universe, "Here I am, and I'm ready." When we take that first small yet monumental step, which is the hardest, the Universe responds.

In my case, my Higher Self responded quickly. The next day, I was in my day treatment program, where I had previously been sitting and frittering away time. But I found out that it offered supported employment. This was a program in which counselors worked with people with mental illness to help them to find employment. I signed up right away.

Taking that first small step didn't mean that I would instantly become the self that I am today, but it was a matter of making the first choice towards my ultimate recovery and alignment with Spirit. In putting on that suit, I was declaring to my Highest Self that I was not the walking dead person that I believed myself to be. It was as if my whole body had been ensconced in plaster, and putting on the suit was making the first cracks in it: cracks which would ultimately lead to freedom.

At that point, I didn't have a full plan laid out. I just knew that I wanted a better life than I had, and that was enough. Hope is a powerful feeling: it can give a person wings.

I encourage you to take this moment and just dream. Believe me, if a deeply depressed mental patient can find something to dream about, so can you. The dream that comes into your mind may seem small and insignificant, but it's not. We will talk more about how to dream in the next chapter, but in the meantime, just allow yourself to envision a life that is different than what you have now.

Imagine a life where you are unstuck. Imagine a life where you are free: free from self-doubt, free from incessant inner criticism. Imagine a life where things go right most of the time for you because you are aligned with All That Is.

Now think of the minutest step towards that life. It might be picking your dirty clothes off the floor and hanging them up. It might be taking a shower. Whatever you do, visualize your dream life as you are doing it. Think of the significance that this baby step can have on your life. If you can't get there yet, that's OK; take the step anyway. The Universe responds to action. You will find that after you act, you will hear a small whisper, which is the Joyful Highway giving you the next step. Remember, a body in motion stays in motion.

Learn How to Dream

While I was living in supported housing with no job, I started attending a day treatment center for people with mental illness. "Program," as they called this day treatment center, was really a misnomer. When I think of programs, I think of structure, order, and most importantly, things to do. Program in reality was a group of about eleven of us who sat downstairs. Upstairs were the people who had been coming to program for years. They had illnesses that had progressed over time, and they were not functioning in society at all.

I suppose that could have been my path as well, but I was still so young that they put me in the group that met downstairs. This was the group that got "therapy," versus the upstairs crowd, who were all a part of "clerical." To this day, I do not know what that group did under the guise of job training skills. Most of them seemed to be rocking back and forth in their chairs muttering to themselves, and staff barely interacted with them at all.

Downstairs, "therapy" consisted of being given handouts from a workbook on depression photocopied by an eager intern, probably with optimism that these sheets of paper were going to be *the thing* to help us get our lives back on track.

On one particular day after my suit experience, our social work intern came bouncing in. She was a thin blonde with way too much mascara and way too much enthusiasm for my taste. She was attending Rutgers for a master's in social work, and this was her current internship placement.

"Hi everyone!" she said in a high-pitched tone that was shrill to my ears. I rolled my eyes internally, but some of my peers in the program were not quite as subtle. One person from group, a young man who always wore a hoodie, had his head down on the table and pretended to sleep—a vain attempt at keeping our own personal Marcia Brady out.

But the intern, whose real name was Barbie, was undeterred. "Guess what?" she said enthusiastically. "Today we are going to talk about your dreams." She turned around to the white board and wrote the word "dreams" on it with big bubbly letters that took up half of the space available. I swear that if dreams were spelled with an "I," she would have dotted it with a heart.

Barbie, who in my opinion was better suited to be a kindergarten teacher than a social worker, continued: "I have a very special worksheet for you today, and I can't wait to give it out."

Ugh. Did she drink Pepto Bismol just for the bubblegum flavor? A few of us groaned, and the rest of the downstairs crew looked away. We knew about worksheets, and after months in this room, we knew of their inefficacy. I wanted to run upstairs and move along with the supported employment group, but this was my scheduled time for this group, so I had no choice. I was stuck with Little Miss Happy and her pep rally.

But, remember, this was post–baby step number one for me, and the Universe had something different in store for today.

Barbie handed out the worksheet quickly, licking her finger to separate the pages. Her long, French manicured nails scratched the paper as she went.

"I'm handing these pages out to you upside down on *purpose*," Barbie said. "No peeking until everybody gets one."

Double ugh. Not only were we humiliated by the fact that we were in a day treatment program for people with mental illness, we were being treated like elementary school kids. Still, I played along and didn't flip my paper over. I didn't want Barbie to cry.

When everyone had a piece of paper, Barbie said, like a cheerleader, "OK, it's time to look!" Clearly she was very satisfied with herself, and I have to admit, I was curious at this point.

On the other side of the paper was not the usual worksheet. It was just a question. In big, bold typed letters that took up the page, it said, "What would you do if you KNEW you wouldn't fail?"

"Now," Barbie said, handing out lined paper, "write." With that, she moved her seat to the corner of the room and began filing her nails, looking very satisfied with herself.

Sometimes the messengers of the Creative Intelligence come in unlikely forms. As much as I don't want to admit it, on that day, Barbie became my messenger.

Ever since my diagnosis with bipolar disorder at age eighteen, my life felt like one failure after another: failed relationships, failed classes, and failed jobs were all I could remember. But now I was being asked to dream, so dream I did.

I thought back to the time when I was a kid and thought about what I had loved to do then. My childhood was a very happy one. I had two loving parents, Dad had a stable job, we were economically thriving, and I did well in school. I also had a lot of nice friends.

Suddenly I remembered something: When I was a little girl, I spent a lot of time in the basement. There I would line up all my dolls in two rows, facing the blackboard that my mother had hung there for me. I would study for my tests by teaching my dolls the school lesson of that day. This was not only my key to getting good grades, it was when I felt most engaged.

A flash of hope came over me again, and I began to write. For the first time, I knew what I wanted for my life. I wanted to be a great educator.

So this is my simple advice about dreaming and daring to dream. Try this exercise for yourself. Write or type on a big piece of paper the words, "What would you do if you knew you would not fail?" Next, get into a peaceful place. You might do this by meditating, or if you are not a meditator, go for a peaceful walk in nature. Really try to clear your head and connect to the Source in whatever way makes the most sense to you. Don't think about the question as you are in this meditative state. You've already put the question out to the Universe just by writing it down on paper.

When you have finished with the meditation, start to consider the question: what would *you* do if you knew you couldn't fail? I find that when I ask my clients this question, the first thing that slaps them in the face is their fear. They say things like, "The thing I would do is stupid," or, "This is a crazy idea, but . . ." This is *normal*. I cannot emphasize this enough. People who are stuck aren't the best dreamers, and they let their self-defeatism get the better of them. You must push past this, and label it for what it is: fear.

Once you have identified the fear, the next step is to feel the fear but think about the dream anyway. You will be assaulted by all the reasons why you can't do what you want to do. This is also normal. Try to push past this too. Get underneath the fear, and really consider the question. Remember, failure is off the table. For the purposes of this exercise, pretend that no matter what you try, you *will* succeed. Does anything come up for you? The thing that sounds so unbelievable, but there is a piece of your heart that really wants to try it—that's your thing.

Now I want you to let yourself dream about this thing, and I have some follow-up questions. Is this thing that you want to do something that makes the time pass quickly when you are doing it? Is it something that you feel like you are guided by a Higher Force while you are doing it? Does the final product feel like it is yours, or is it divinely inspired in some way? Does the thing you are doing benefit the greater good? Does it bring something to the world that is your unique expression of who you are? If so, you are on the right track.

You see, the Law That Guides All Things wants you to do something in this life that is uniquely yours. There is something that you do better than anyone else in the world, and if you want to contribute to the planet and have a meaningful life, you *must* find it. It must not be solely for the money. Money is important, but if you are doing something just for the money, you are not in line with your highest purpose.

Now let's say that nothing is coming to you in this exercise. This does not mean that you do not have a purpose. It means that you are blocked. That's OK. I had an important question that I needed to ask myself to get the ball rolling. Ask yourself, what did I enjoy doing as a child?

I asked this question at a seminar that I was giving last week, and someone said, "I liked riding my hot wheels. What can you do with that?" I asked this gentleman more questions, and it turns out that it translated to now, when he enjoyed taking road trips in his car. "So?" he said. "That's not my vocation. I'm a therapist." I then asked him what he liked about his job. "Well," he said, "it's all about the journey."

"Aha," I said. "You are still metaphorically riding those hot wheels, but your journey now is with your clients, and it's a journey within."

You may have to think abstractly like this, but it's in there. We all have a talent, we all have passions, and we all have something that we can do better than anyone else in the world when we put our own unique spin on it.

Don't Tell Anyone Your Dream...Yet

After group, it was time for supported employment, which was a program to help people with mental illness find jobs. I had high hopes for this—that somehow I would be able to finally bring my plan of becoming a great educator into fruition. The leader of the group was Marsha, a woman in her mid-fifties. She had short, dyed, honey-brown hair and always wore suits, which was unusual at program. Perhaps she was trying to model employment-worthy behavior.

I had had an intake with Marsha, but I wasn't quite sure about my goals. But today I was going to tell her all about my idea. I couldn't wait to get started.

Yet before I could get a word in, Marsha walked into the room excitedly. "Emily," she said, "I have made two really great connections for you for possible job opportunities, and I know that you are going to be pleased."

"Wow," I said, a little surprised. I hadn't yet told Marsha of my new goals, so how was she able to make connections for me?

"*Em*-ily," she said again with great emphasis on the first syllable, "put on your makeup and bring in your best clothes, because you are going to be interviewing for two great part-time jobs. The first is as a grocery bagger at Stop & Shop. The second is as a waitress at Friendly's. Aren't you thrilled?"

I was *not* thrilled at all. Don't get me wrong: it wasn't that I thought myself above either job. It was just that I was a college graduate and wanted a job that was commensurate with my interests and skill set. In her offer of places to interview, I could feel some great stigma. To Marsha, I was a mental patient. She didn't know that I was in the top 4 percent of my high school graduating class or that I went to Rutgers on full academic scholarship and, despite bipolar disorder, managed to graduate with a good GPA. Nor did she seem to care. She also didn't seem to care about my vocational interests and goals. Besides, I am the world's worst grocery bagger. I break eggs and I have no spatial perception, so I can't maximize the bag's potential, and I wind up wasting bags. I would have lost that job in two days.

This is when I made a major mistake. "I want to be a teacher," I said.

Marsha made a face as if she had just sucked on a lemon. "Emily," she said in a way that made me momentarily despise my name, "that's just not possible for you. How are you going to take care of students and manage a classroom when you struggle to care for yourself?"

I knew that "struggle to care for yourself" was a euphemism. What she really meant was, "How can you take care of students when you have a mental illness?"

This was not the last time during my vocational journey that I would get a message like this, but this one stands out in my mind because of how she said it. Marsha had no hope for me, so I had little hope for her ability to help me.

This brings me to the next key to becoming your Highest Self: don't tell everyone about your dream right away. I had a great habit of doing this. When I had a decision to make, like a statistician, I surveyed all my close allies, and in Marsha's case some not-so-close people as well, to figure out what I should do. This is not trusting the Universe at all. It's the ultimate attempt at trying to control things. It's saying, "Universe, I don't believe that you can bring me what I need, so I'm going to ask everyone I know what they think that I should do instead and make my choices based on that."

True positive choices about life can only be made through the Universal Law that guides all things. If the thing you want to do is for the greater good and can also bring you happiness, I believe the Higher Essence will bring it to you. If not, it won't. Simple as that. Humans can see such a small sliver of the Universe that they don't have the best perspective to advise. They don't have enough information, because they don't know the infinite possibilities available to you or what will truly make you happy and bring the greatest benefit for the world. And neither do you.

For this reason, if you tell everyone your dreams too early, they are likely to shoot them down. In my case, that made logical sense. I had just come out of my twelfth hospitalization and had almost been institutionalized for good. *Logically*, I was struggling to care for myself. Logically, it *should* have been difficult for me to be a teacher. But the Universe doesn't do logic. It does callings.

A calling is something that you are meant to do. I believe that it is a contract with the Higher Mind that you make before you are even born: you decide what you will do to bring good to this world. Yes, this is my belief, but it's not original. Many of the great thinkers that have walked the planet have said something similar.

A dream is a tender, fragile thing. If you tell people about your dreams too soon, their opinions may dishearten you. Get going on your dreams first, telling yourself, "The Universe has my back." Later, when people see you doing the thing that is your dream, they may still criticize, but you are less likely to hear them or take it to heart. You will be too busy doing what you love to notice.

⚬━━🎋 Key 13

Develop the Ability to Bounce

Back in supported employment, I decided not to listen to Marsha and find my own opportunities. I wrote my own résumé by copying a format that I found through Google. I wrote a cover letter much the same way. I took a part-time job as a filing clerk in a law office where my friend Alisa was working as a paralegal. She got me the job.

But my skills as a worker were still not developed. After years of being in and out of a psych hospital, I didn't have much time to develop adult skills. I did my laundry and cooked occasionally, but that was about it. I lost the job in two months.

Undeterred, I continued applying to jobs. Although I wanted to be an educator, my college degree was in English, so I lacked the credentials to teach. But I still wanted to work in the field of education, so I was applying to jobs in tutoring centers. Finally, I thought to network. I had a sorority sister who was a director at a tutoring center. I decided to send her my résumé, and sure enough, I secured an interview for a job as a full-time assistant director of the Learning Center. This role was administrative and involved supervising the tutors. It was a great fit for my interests.

I remember the interview very clearly. I first met with a regional director named Giselle. She was a woman of about fifty with long, straight blond hair and long nails. "So tell me about yourself," she started the interview, tapping on the desk with her pen.

"Crap," I thought. Dad, who luckily was a recruiter, prepared me for this question, but I still hated it. It conjured up images of me at my worst with my mental health struggles. I thought of straitjackets I was strapped into, police chasing me, and then that awful click of the door behind me each time I was locked away in the psych hospital. This was my identity, but obviously I couldn't tell this to Giselle. I would have to do my best acting.

"Well," I started, "I majored in English at Rutgers University, and I have a real passion for educating today's youth."

"Yes," I thought, "this sounds good." I began to smile and relax and let my true self come out. "I took a course in education in college, and I got to do some student teaching in a fourth-grade classroom. This was a wonderful experience for me!"

This was all true. I did have a semester where I thought about applying to the graduate program in education at Rutgers. It was my best semester, and I loved every minute of working with the kids.

From that answer, I knew that I had Giselle. When I am passionate about something, I can be quite persuasive, and I let the passion carry me, not my anxiety. When we were finished, Giselle sent in the wife of the owner of the company. She was lovely, and they offered me the job just a few days later.

Unfortunately, the Learning Center was not a good fit for me, although I gained some good experience there and learned about what I liked and disliked in a job. My boss was a morbidly obese woman who swore like a truck driver and yelled with the ferocity of a tornado when things weren't going her way. And I was a big part of things not going her way.

I had many things working against me on this job. First, my medicine made me so tired that I could not get up for work on time, which looked quite unprofessional. Remember, I hadn't had the ability to develop any workplace skills whatsoever. I was basically flying blind as a bat (minus the sound waves for direction). And while I enjoyed supervising the tutors and even occasionally got to tutor kids (whom I loved), I was terrible at the administrative tasks. At that time my mind was still not sharp enough to pay attention to detail.

"Emily," my boss shrieked one day, "look at this report!" Her eyes were popping out of her large head. "You have callously filled out the report again!" I looked at the report. I had rushed through it and made a lot of mistakes.

"Linda," I said, "*callous* means that I maliciously filled out the report, trying to mess up, which I did not. I think the word that you are looking for is *careless*." Not the best way to talk to one's angry boss.

Her face turned crimson, and she continued shrieking. "Whatever!" she said angrily. "You are skating on thin ice around here, Emily. You better be careful, and not just with reports."

Sweat trickled down her forehead, and I could see sweat stains under her armpits as she flailed her arms with rage.

I was fired after only nine months on the job. I was horrified at first, but I was determined not to let this experience sink me back into the deep abyss that is depression. I would *not* be a mental patient anymore. I had to keep on moving. By this point, I had moved out of the shared apartment in Freehold and moved in with some girls my age in Belmar, New Jersey. I was terrified about how I would pay my bills and began scouring the Internet for jobs. In the meantime, I got my substitute teacher license to bring in money, and I began subbing.

Subbing turned out to be great for me. It was a nice supplement to my unemployment checks, and I had enough to live on. I was in the classroom again and felt I had come home. I adored the kids, especially the fourth and fifth graders. They understood my sense of humor. These were "my people," I thought.

While I was still applying to jobs, I got another idea. I remembered my envy that one of my sorority sisters had gotten into Columbia University's Teachers College in our senior year at Rutgers. I knew that it was a long shot for me. I had good grades, but I also had a ton of W's on my transcript, which stood for "withdrawal." In school, I was in and out of the psych hospital so much that I often had to abruptly stop classes for treatment. Luckily, I had partnered with the most compassionate dean of disabilities, Clarence Shive, who helped me to pull out of the classes with a W and not a failing grade. These W's did not hurt my GPA, but I thought that my transcript looked suspect nonetheless.

I don't know how I had the confidence to apply at all. I remember poring over the course catalogue, looking at the cover, which had Teachers College's beautiful cathedral on it. Looking back, I don't think that it truly was confidence that helped me hastily pull together my application just days before the deadline. There was something pulling me, nudging me in the direction of Teachers College that was beyond sheer ambition. It was my passion, my bliss.

As the deadline approached to receive word, I was at the mailbox every day. Finally one day, I saw a business-sized envelope with blue lettering that said "Teachers College." This was it. I prayed for Grace to provide for me. I didn't really know who I was praying to; I just prayed. I guess it was the God that I had learned about in Hebrew school. As I explained earlier, this God rewarded and punished. I prayed that my years of punishment with my mental illness were over and that I'd been good enough to receive this amazing opportunity.

I held my breath as I ripped open the envelope. As I sucked in some air, I closed my eyes, afraid to look. Finally I opened the letter and began reading:

"Dear Ms. Grossman,

Congratulations on your acceptance to the Teaching of English Masters of Arts program at Teachers College..."

I didn't read the rest. My hands shook so violently that you could see the paper flapping around. I did it, and I was feeling elated—and terrified.

In my survey of allies and even some enemies, it was unanimous: I should not go. Different people had different reasons for this. Some shared the sentiments of Marsha, the supported employment counselor: how could a woman with mental illness take care of her students? Others were more fearful about the $60,000 loan I'd have to take out. With my track record of getting fired from jobs, how would I ever repay it? These discussions were enough to put deep fear in me. I had yet to understand how to trust the Universe. Still, I wasn't ready to pull the plug completely. Ultimately, I decided to defer for a year to try to work and save some money for school if I was to go at all.

Just days later, one of my online applications for a job resulted in a phone interview for a job at an SAT tutoring company. In fact, it was the very company that had tutored me for the SATs. In the face-to-face interview, I turned on the old charisma again.

"I'm the poster child for this company. I was tutored by you for my SAT's and saw a tremendous rise in my scores. I really believe in your organization." And just like that, I had my second job after college.

Yet I had similar struggles with my residue of mental health symptoms. I was always tired from my medication. I even fell asleep at my desk a couple of times. I was hardly a stellar employee. The part of the job that I did love, though, was teaching SAT classes. I had a blast doing this. Again I was fired within nine months, although my boss was compassion- ate enough to let me continue to do the SAT teaching.

Again, I took it hard. I felt like it reflected who I was as a person. I had a hard time separating what was illness from what was intrinsic to my character. I felt like a failure, but again I started to apply to new jobs. I began to see a pattern.

Fearing that my life was going to be one vicious cycle of getting and losing jobs that weren't interesting, I thought about Mrs. Collins and following my bliss again. I didn't know why, but I knew in my heart that I needed to go back to school. I would see later why this was such an important life choice.

No question that this was not the most externally successful period in my life. Yet looking back on it, I do see the triumph of it all. I was learning to bounce. No longer was I viewing life setbacks as a reason to go back into the hospital, which at times had become my second home. As difficult as this period was, I was developing a new set of coping strategies to tolerate my discomfort and keep my depression from deepening into suicidal thoughts. This was largely due to the help of my therapist Sherrie, to whom I am forever indebted.

The next key in attaining your Highest Life State is developing an ability to bounce. I think back to those small bouncing balls that one could buy in vending machines at Kmart when I was a kid in the 1980s. I remember begging my mother for a quarter, placing it in the machine's silver slot, twisting the metal lever, and then waiting expectantly to see what color I would get, always hoping for the hot pink one or the one that was clear with gold glitter.

It's an interesting thing about those little bouncing balls. I discovered very soon in my youth that if I sat on the floor and bounced the ball, it would not bounce back very high. I realized that the ball needed to fall from a greater height to make a high bounce back. So I stood on the stairs, threw the ball over the banister, and watched with delight how high it would bounce.

I believe that I am just like this bouncing ball, and so are you. If you drop me from a great height, I will definitely fall, but watch out, because I will also bounce back very high. You too have that capacity. That's the way the Universe created you. When you have a great fall, you don't have to stay stuck. You can bounce. And the ability to bounce is what matters far more than the fall.

When I was a child, my Grandma Trudy once pulled me close to her. Grandma was an elfin type with short, curly orange hair that she dyed herself, with little success. What she lacked in hair coloring skills she made up for in wisdom. She delivered it in the form of clichés, but they were usually accurate ones. On this day, she looked me right in the eyes.

"Emily," she said, her impish nature falling away for a moment as she took a more serious tone, "life is like a roller coaster. Sometimes you are up and sometimes you are down, but remember in the downs that you will always go back up."

I took this advice very seriously. Even though in college, I didn't know how to bounce, I held onto Grandma Trudy's words, and a little piece of me knew that she was right. It would get better. It had to.

So if you are struggling right now in your life, cultivate the ability to bounce. Despite all of my setbacks, I didn't give up; I just kept on bouncing. I know that you can do it too. Successful people don't have everything go right all the time. They have resilience—the ability to bounce. They look at setbacks and find opportunity in them. In Buddhism, we talk of turning obstacles into opportunities: every setback can lead to spiritual growth that ultimately gives one momentum to overcome the obstacle. When I started looking at life this way, I became free of perfectionism, because I knew that my "failures" were truly lessons that would bring me to the next level spiritually. I also became free of self-pity because I stopped saying, "Why me?" every time I was confronted by a challenge. Today, when an obstacle hits, I refresh my determination to overcome it and get moving to solve the problem. Successful people may make it look easy, but if you really talk to them, you will find that their lives too were a series of ups and downs. Here's to bouncing.

Plant Seeds

It was the summer of 2003, and I was back at the psychiatrist's office to get my medication renewed. I was very bored
while I was waiting for my psychiatrist, who was chronically
late. I looked at the coffee table, which was cluttered with
magazines, when something caught my attention. I'm not
sure why I picked it up, but it was a newsletter for the local
chapter of NAMI: the National Alliance on Mental Illness. It
was known as NAMI Monmouth, because it was headquar-
tered in Monmouth County, New Jersey.

I thumbed through the newsletter a bit skeptically. I wasn't
one for groups, and most of the newsletter listed support
groups that were being held locally. But something pushed
me to read on. The newsletter was black-and-white and about
four pages long. On the last page in the lower right-hand corner was an advertisement that said, "Want to Tell Your Mental Health Recovery Story?" and gave the phone number of

a man named Mark. I was intrigued. I had always wanted to share my story and see if it could benefit others.

I called Mark that night, and luckily he picked up the phone on the first ring. "Hello?" he said.

"Hi, my name is Emily, and I saw your advertisement in the NAMI newsletter about training people to tell their recovery stories. Are you still doing it?"

"Yes," Mark replied, "and there's an information session tomorrow. Why don't you come?"

"Great!" I said. I got the address from Mark and anxiously awaited the next day's events.

In the car on the way to the info session, I got a surge of energy. I felt that tingling sensation, and something intuitively told me that I was about to experience some magic. I was right about this, but I wouldn't see it unfold for many years.

The info session itself wasn't a monumental experience. I met Mark, his wife, Paula and some other prospective speakers, which was nice, and I signed up to go to the training for a program called In Our Own Voice (IOOV), where people told their mental health recovery stories. This was also quite nice, but that was about it.

Training would start in a few weeks, so I made sure that I had the times in my calendar and left the meeting largely unaffected. I was even a bit disappointed. I was constantly looking for signs that I was on my path towards the right career, and on this particular evening I hadn't seen any. I wrote off the feeling I had gotten in my car as just a coincidence and left it at that.

The day arrived when I was going to be participating in the IOOV training. I walked into the conference room of the

Sheraton Hotel, where the training was going to be held, with no expectations. I really liked the people that I had met at the info session, but again, I was looking for concrete signs, and I really hadn't gotten any.

Mark and Paula were there, and they gave me my name tag, a navy blue folder, and some index cards. I took my seat and began to flip through the materials inside the folder. When it was time to start, Mark came to the center of the room and introduced us to a man who was going to be our trainer. As soon as the trainer, Robin, took the floor, I was captivated by him. He was a man of about sixty with gray hair, and he was dressed very elegantly in a navy blue suit with a red handkerchief in the right pocket and a red tie. He walked with a redwood cane and was quite professional in appearance and manner.

"Hello, everyone," Robin began. "One of my favorite things to do is to teach this course. You see, I was diagnosed with schizophrenia in the 1940s, well before good medication came out. My doctor worked very hard with me from a young age to help me stay on track. He did a form of therapy that was a precursor to cognitive behavioral therapy. I responded extremely well. Also, although my behaviors were sometimes strange in high school, a group of the popular kids took me under their wing, and this helped my self-esteem very much. I was able to not only graduate from college but get my MBA. I ended up becoming a high-level executive at several different Fortune 500 companies. I have recently retired, and I'm now writing my memoir."

I was blown away. This was the first time that I was hearing the story of someone with mental illness who had "made it" and come out the other side into a successful life. I really wanted what Robin had. I was inspired. I had been waiting years to hear the message that he gave that day. This was my sign.

In the five-day workshop, I worked hard to learn to tell my own story. The IOOV team had cleverly broken the training down into five sections, each accompanied by a video of people living in recovery who spoke of their experience. The five sections started with "The Dark Days" and chronicled the journey through "Recovery." We wrote each section on an index card and rehearsed the sections in front of the rest of the group.

When the training was done, I was on fire with enthusiasm and couldn't wait to start. I was booked right away to do an IOOV talk at Monmouth College, a private college in West Long Branch, New Jersey. I remember that talk well. I was very nervous beforehand, and I prayed that I would be able to touch just one person in the room. Since it was my first talk, I was paired up with another presenter, Jill.

Throughout the talk, I felt as though the Universe was working through me, giving me the words to say. It was a sublime, otherworldly experience. I was in my body, but there were moments where it didn't feel that way. I felt as though I were floating a few feet above, looking in on myself, and I liked what I was seeing. For the first time in a long time, I felt like myself. After the talk, several people came over to me and said that I had inspired them. I hadn't known joy like that in some time.

In my car afterward, I opened up my black flip cell phone and called Mark. "How'd it go?" he asked expectantly.

"Mark, it was just great. I feel like I've found my passion and my calling. How do I do this for a living?" I asked enthusiastically.

Mark laughed, and then said, "You don't! If someone could make a living doing this, I would have figured out how a long time ago. There just aren't jobs like this out there."

One would think that after hearing something like this, I would have been totally deflated. And for a moment or two, I really was. But I'm a fighter. I don't give up when I know that I'm on to something, so I tucked this dream away for a while and let it incubate. I also sent my dream out into the Universe that night. I knew that the Higher Mind hears our deepest longings, and that some way, somehow, I *must* turn this dream into a reality.

The next key to becoming your Higher Self is to plant seeds. People who are doing wonderful things with their lives didn't just snap their fingers and get there. They had to do a few things to build to that point, and one of them was to plant seeds in the Universe with their intentions. Every dream begins with a seed planted. Every dream begins with a declaration to the Higher Source about what a person wants to do. The Universe does eventually hear you, even if the people in your life don't.

When I was speaking about my mental health recovery, I felt alive in a way that I hadn't since I was a small child. Everything became vivid and clear. I didn't have to think carefully to choose my words; they just came. While I was speaking, I was totally in the moment. I knew in that instant that I wanted to use my life to share my mental health recovery story and inspire others. I just didn't know how to get there.

I had done a lot of reading about setting intentions. You don't have to know how something is going to end up. You just have to set an intention that it will, and slowly, if it is the right dream for you to pursue for your happiness and for the good of the world, the Higher Mind will work on the details.

Setting intentions is what I mean by planting seeds. In Buddhism, we talk a lot about "making determinations." This is how we tell the Mystic Law what we hope will happen in our lives. We don't get all of our determinations, but as I said earlier, the ones that are for the greater good usually materialize.

In Nichiren Buddhism—the school of Buddhism that I follow—we chant *nam myoho renge kyo*. *Renge* means *lotus flower*, which is the only flower that both blossoms and seeds at the same time. This represents the idea that when you make a determination, you are planting a seed, and the blossom from that seed is already manifested out in the Universe; you just need to pull it to you. I pull my intentions toward me by chanting, but if chanting is not right for you, other practices can work. Some people might do a more traditional type of meditation. Some may go for a walk in nature or perform some type of ritual. It is important that you get your mind quiet and then release your intentions. This is a practice that Deepak Chopra calls "going into the gap." You need to be really connected to your Higher Power in order to plant a seed of your intentions.

Once the seed is planted, I believe that the Greater Consciousness scans all the possibilities for your life, which are infinite, and assesses which seeds should blossom based on which ones are truly meant for your happiness and the good of the world, and which ones are not. We can see so little of the Universe with our human minds that we cannot fathom which desires are best to be fulfilled and which aren't. Usually when I don't manifest a desire, it's because there was something infinitely better waiting for me. Be patient with your Higher Power. It will bring you the best things for your happiness. Please trust that.

⚷— Key 15

Find HP: Part 2

Remember when I prayed to the God of my youth to find a practice like the one that Deepak Chopra wrote about? Well, for years, nothing miraculous happened to me spiritually at all. In fact, I went through an inferno of the spirit which was so intense that I doubted the presence of a Higher Power at all.

Then, in the fall of 2005, it was time to go to Teachers College. As my taxi pulled up to the front of the new dorm where I would be living, on 120th Street and Amsterdam Avenue in New York City, I felt a surge of adrenaline like what I had felt after reading Chopra's book. I was now officially a student at Columbia University and also officially $60,000 in debt. I chose to focus on the former.

Getting out of the cab with my things, I stood up straighter than I had in a long time. I had confidence again. It was a shallow confidence created only by my current status as an Ivy

League student, but I hadn't had anything to feel confident about in so long that it felt really good. As I said earlier, when I thought about going to Columbia, I was nudged so hard by the Universe that its power practically drove me there itself. In a few weeks I would learn why.

Soon after my arrival, I was working on a group project for a class with my new friend, Nicole. Nicole always had a lightness of spirit to her. Today she bounced cheerfully into the small room in the library. "Hey, Em," she said energetically and sat down.

"Hey," I responded. Nicole's face radiated with a loving, compassionate energy. She never wore makeup, but she didn't need it: her essence was that bright.

Then something came out of my mouth that surprised us both. "Nicole, one day I'm going to move to Southern California and become a Buddhist."

Nicole's tiny mouth opened wide as her jaw dropped.

"What?" I said, thinking that she thought I had lost it.

"I'm from Southern California, and I'm a Buddhist," she said, "and there's a meeting tonight. You *need* to come!" Nicole was practically chirping at this point.

I thought about it only for a split second. We were so aligned in that moment that I made an instant decision. "Of course I'll come," I said, sure that this was the right choice.

I don't remember too much about that first meeting except that I arrived late. By the time I got there, they were showing a video about world peace. "This is interesting," I thought, but to be honest, the meeting didn't make much of an impression on me. I had a long way to go before world peace would become a priority.

I returned home feeling a bit disappointed. When Nicole brought up the meeting, I felt that the Divine was guiding me to go. Yet I hadn't really experienced anything otherworldly.

The next day our dorm had a get-together. I was curious to see if I would meet anyone new, especially a man. Men seemed to be few and far between at school. I walked in and saw Nicole right away.

"Emily, there's someone that I want you to meet," she said, chirping again, and leading me in the direction of one of the only men in the room. He was of medium height with a crew cut, dark hair, and equally dark eyes. He was wearing a sports jacket with jeans and indoor soccer shoes and talking casually to one of the other people in our dorm.

"This is my friend Gonzalo, from undergrad. He's engaged to my friend Mafe," Nicole said.

"Hi," Gonzalo said with a thick Argentinian accent. "Nice to meet you, Emily. I heard that you were at our Buddhist meeting yesterday—so sorry that I could not be there to meet you then."

He spoke as if it was part of the plan for us both to be at that meeting and that he had not held up his end of the commitment. His sincerity, combined with charisma, made me hang on every word as he spoke. Although we had only just met, I felt I had known him for a lifetime. I didn't know if I believed in reincarnation at that point, but in that moment, if you had told me that we had been friends in a past lifetime, I would have absolutely believed you.

"Nicole and I went to Soka University, which is the university that is run by the Soka Gakkai International. This is the name of the Buddhist organization to which we belong.

Soka Gakkai means 'value creation society.' We practice a form of Buddhism called Nichiren Buddhism, which originated in Japan."

Gonzalo continued talking about Nichiren Buddhism and its philosophy for quite some time. I was captivated. I loved the theory of attaining world peace by helping each individual to become truly happy. I loved the idea that Nichiren Buddhists were taught to cherish each person. I believe we spoke for a good hour, and at that point it was getting late. But I knew that Gonzalo would have an important place in my life and that I could look to him for some serious spiritual guidance.

A few weeks passed, and I didn't see Gonzalo. It was late September by the time I saw him again. "Emily," he said, greeting me like an old friend, "the San Gennaro Festival is tonight, and a few of us are going. Would you like to join?"

"I really would," I said. I had been hoping I'd have another opportunity to speak to this gentle Buddhist with the lovely accent. I wanted to learn more about Buddhism, and I was hoping I would have an opportunity to do so at the festival.

San Gennaro is a festival that takes place in the early fall every year in New York's Little Italy. Restaurants throughout this area throw their doors open and serve delicious Italian food of all kinds. In addition, there are street venders selling everything from fresh mozzarella to sausages and peppers. For the kids, there are games and rides. The colorful and scrumptious festival goes on for blocks and blocks, and the streets are closed for days.

As we were walking towards the subway, an undergraduate named Molly, who also practiced with the Soka Gakkai, asked Gonzalo, "Have you ever tried to go a few days without chanting? Isn't it awful?"

"Chanting?" I said inquisitively. "I didn't see any chanting at the meeting that I went to."

"Really?" Gonzalo asked, looking surprised. "That's the whole basis of the practice."

"I was a little late," I replied, blushing a bit from embarrassment. "Maybe I missed the chanting?"

Gonzalo laughed. "I'm sure that was the case, because we always start the meetings by chanting for a bit."

Gonzalo and Molly then began to describe the chanting to me. They told me that in Nichiren Buddhism, they chant the Japanese words *nam myoho renge kyo*. Roughly translated, these words mean: "I pledge my devotion to the Mystic Law of Cause and Effect through sound." The Mystic Law is the energy that guides all things. It's the force that makes the plants grow, makes eggs hatch into birds, and makes mothers give birth to their children. In Nichiren Buddhism, it is the Higher Power, which is found within. Cause and effect is a key of the Mystic Law. It basically means that for every action, there is a reaction. When you do something good in the world, something positive is bound to manifest, and the same is true for negative actions, or causes, as we call them.

As much as I was enjoying the festival, the whole time I really wanted to go home and learn to chant, which Gonzalo and Nicole had promised we could do. When we got back to our dorm, Nicole, Gonzalo, and I went into Nicole's room. There was a black box with two doors, which I later learned was called a *butsudan*, or altar. Nicole turned on a light and opened the two doors. What was inside was awe-inspiring.

"This is the *gohonzon*, Emily," Nicole said after she ceremoniously swung the doors open. "It's a pictorial depiction of enlightenment." I didn't know what that even meant, but I was mesmerized. The gohonzon was a white scroll with black Japanese lettering all over it. Surrounding the writing was a beautiful green and white design. It hung from a ribbon on a hook, which sat in the middle of the butsudan.

I had so many questions, but before I could ask any of them, Gonzalo came behind me. "Ring the bell, Nicole. Let's chant."

Slowly Gonzalo, Nicole, and I chanted in unison. I didn't love it at first. It was hard to pronounce the words, and I think I was hoping to be struck by enlightenment in that first session, which didn't happen. But I felt so connected to Nicole and Gonzalo and so grateful for their sincerity and the care they were taking of me that I vowed to continue, at least for a little while, to see what was in store.

I believe that finding your Higher Power, or HP, as it's called in the Twelve Step programs, is one of the most important things that you can do in order to become your Highest Self. Most people spend hours in front of the television living a fantasy life, yet they rarely give five minutes a day to enlarging their spiritual life. And many times that's all it takes to begin to connect.

I can see the atheists and agnostics coming to a screeching halt here. They may think, "I've been successful in life without God." I guess that all depends upon your belief about success. For me, a successful life is one that transcends ego and attachment. It is a life where one learns to be happy in the moment, without waiting for that new job, new car, or new partner to make you happy. There's only one thing that can make one happy, and that is oneself. Success is a life in which one discovers their highest purpose and learns to serve others. To make any of this possible, one needs a Higher Power to connect to instead of being stuck in self.

I am not suggesting that everyone must have the *same* Higher Power. In this book, you have thus far heard me refer to HP as many different things. I'm not advocating for any one religion or spiritual practice. Buddhism is right for me, but you may have other beliefs that satisfy your questions about the Universe and All That Is. I am suggesting that, as they say in Twelve Step programs, you have a connection to something higher. That is all. It may be nature, it may be love, it may be God or Allah or Jesus or Krishna.

Ego can be a fragile thing to rely upon for positive feelings. One minute you feel elated because your boss gave you a raise, and the next, you feel deflated because a man or woman didn't return your affection. It's extremely burdensome to live this way, and it takes a ton of energy. Connecting to an HP is not giving up your power; it's acknowledging that you are human and flawed and that there is a perfect energy that guides all things and can guide you too. In Buddhism, when we chant, we believe that we are connecting to that Higher Force, and it is helping us to bring out our Highest Self, which we call our "Buddha nature." Many other practices have similar beliefs.

No matter how you connect with your HP, be it through prayer, meditation, yoga, or other rituals, it takes a lot of the pressure off you. No longer do you feel that you must control everything. The law of the Universe is omniscient and omnipotent; we are not. But when this law works through us, we gain our power.

In his prose poem "Desiderata," Max Ehrmann writes, "You are a child of the universe, no less than the trees and the stars; you have a right to be here. And whether or not it is clear to you, no doubt the universe is unfolding as it should."

Whenever I find my ego trying to control things, I remember this quote. I do have a right to be in the Universe, but not to control it. I take comfort in the fact that Higher Force is always at work in my life, and that whether I understand it or not, there is a flow and a natural order to things, and they will work out in the best way for me and for the Highest Good. The more I believe this, the more things do work out, because I am a cocreator of life with the Mystic Law.

$\text{o---}\!\!\!\text{---}$ Key 16

Ride the Waves

I chanted to get a job right after graduate school teaching sixth or seventh grade. Manifesting things is a big part of chanting, and sure enough, during my last months at Teachers College, I was hired by a school district in northern New Jersey to teach seventh grade starting in the fall of 2006.

Chanting had made a major impact on every aspect of my life. The biggest change was that my symptoms of mental illness seemed to fall away. I cannot explain this, but I will say that I knew it was the chanting, because my medication didn't change and I hadn't made any other adjustments that could have resulted in my healing. It seemed that chanting really worked, so I joined the Soka Gakkai International (SGI) and received my own gohonzon, the special scroll in front of which I chanted.

Teaching was a lot harder than I thought it would be. While I loved being up in front of my students and teaching lessons, I learned quickly that this was only part of the job. The other parts, such as catering to the many needs of parents, administrators, and other teachers, were much harder and less desirable.

Something else happened too. It was after class my second year in the classroom, in the fall of 2007. I was thirty years old. This time I was teaching sixth grade. It was a welcome change, as seventh graders tend to test authority a bit more than sixth graders do.

Fifth period had just ended, and I had my lunch break. I would typically eat in my classroom to avoid the teachers' lounge, which I found to have a lot of negative energy and complaining. A student was at the door, and I asked him to come in.

He was one of my favorite students. He was a bit shorter than the other boys and was quite mild-mannered. He always participated in class, raising his hand straight up like an arrow when he knew the answer. He had very curly brown hair, dark eyes, and olive skin. His features on his face were quite small, with a small nose and mouth. Many of the girls in my class had huge crushes on him.

He looked at me intensely, and I could tell by his energy that something was seriously wrong. I had noticed over the past few days that his participation had fallen away and he seemed preoccupied. I was glad that he was approaching me.

"Ms. Grossman," he began with a garbled voice, choking back tears, "my girlfriend just broke up with me the other day. It really hurt."

"I'm so sorry," I said to him. "That sounds like it was really difficult. I know that you really cared about her."

"Yeah," he sniffed, "I don't think I can ever love again like that."

I worked hard not to chuckle at this, but I kept a straight face and a kind demeanor towards him. I really liked him and wanted to make sure that I was as empathetic as possible. When my students came to me with personal problems, I always considered it a gift. It meant that I was doing my job properly, because I was building an atmosphere of trust in my classroom.

"Ms. Grossman," my student continued, "there's something else. It's kind of hard to tell you, but I know I should tell an adult. After my girlfriend broke up with me, I was in such pain, and I didn't know how to get rid of it. So I started cutting myself."

He rolled up his sleeve, and I could see about ten cuts on the back of his forearm. They were relatively superficial, but they were there nonetheless.

Externally, I remained calm, but on the inside it was as if my heart had been torn from my chest. I swallowed hard to compose myself. As I said earlier in the book, when I'm sad, or feeling any intense emotion for that matter, my throat tightens and it's difficult to swallow without feeling soreness.

"I'm so grateful that you shared this with me," I said. "Any thoughts of taking your own life?" I asked.

"No," he said. "I just feel very sad, and I don't know how to get rid of that feeling, so I am cutting myself to release it."

"OK," I said. "I know that it's hard to feel your feelings right now. They must be very intense. But it's important to look for ways to cope that aren't hurting your body. I hope you understand that I have to tell a guidance counselor about this.

I know that you trusted me, but I really cannot keep things like this a secret; otherwise I will get into trouble."

I was going to go on, but the principal came running in, and my student quickly rolled down his sleeve and ran out of the door. "Ms. Grossman, what was that all about?" she said, eyeing me suspiciously.

Mrs. Worthington was a stern woman who had worked in corporate for many years before she became first a teacher and then a principal. She ran our school like a business and tended to micromanage the nontenured teachers, of which I was one. I was terrified of her.

I began to stutter and stammer, not sure how to tell her, although I knew that I had to. "He . . . wa . . . wa . . . was cutting himself because he is sad that his girlfriend broke up with him," I squeaked out.

"Ms. Grossman! You should know better than to get involved in these kinds of issues. That's why we have guidance counselors. When a student comes to you like that, the first thing that you should do is send him to the guidance counselor. A teacher has no place interfering. You aren't trained to understand and help with these kinds of issues! This is very irresponsible of you, and I will have to document your behavior," Mrs. Worthington said, almost shrieking.

Little did she know that I knew a ton about those kinds of issues through my own lived experience. I felt extremely helpless. Our guidance counselors were the ones who had little experience with these issues. They were great at doing people's schedules but less good at the mental health aspect of the job. It wasn't really their fault. Guidance counselors just aren't traditionally trained that way.

This was not the only time that I had students come to me with mental health concerns; it was just the first. In fact, because of my reputation around the school as someone who was into self-help, a lot of the students started coming to me. Each time they did, I received a similar reprimand from my administration. I didn't know what to do.

At the same time, I was struggling outside of the classroom as well. I had been casually dating two different men, both of whom broke off with me at the same time. I took it very personally and viewed it as rejection. I started spiraling quickly into a deep depression. I tried to be proactive and went to my psychiatrist.

"Emily," he said as soon as he saw me, "you look terrible." Dr. Ashrot was a middle-aged man with an arrogant manner. He once told me that when he married his wife, she didn't know that he smoked because he had hidden it from her while they were dating. In any event, he was my psychiatrist, and even though I questioned some of his ethics and values, I needed a psychiatrist, so I stayed with him.

I was living in Hoboken at the time, and Dr. Ashrot's office was just down the turnpike in Bayonne. His office was rather large, and he had lots of stuffed, mounted fish that he had caught over the years hanging on the pale blue walls.

"Emily," he went on, "you are too depressed at this point. If you want to continue working with me, we *must* change your medicine. There's this medicine called lithium for bipolar. Ever heard of it?'

I began to shudder. Lithium, a salt that has helped people with bipolar disorder, is an older mood stabilizer known for producing weight gain in some people. I did not want this.

I was hoping to meet the right gentleman to marry, and I didn't want to struggle with my figure, which had been slender and fit.

"I'm not taking that!" I said with a determined tone. I had to let Dr. Ashrot know that I meant business. "It will make me gain weight."

Dr. Ashrot half smiled in a way that emphasized his arrogance. "OK," he said. "Then I won't see you anymore."

I thought about this. I was in a deep depression again and clinging to my job with all my might, and I couldn't let myself go all the way back to the way I was before. Also, in my depression, I didn't have the energy to start calling around to find a new doctor. This may sound lazy, but having depression and trying to do even simple daily tasks is like trying to run the marathon with concrete on your legs: things feel nearly impossible. Because of all of this, I decided to follow Dr. Ashrot's advice and take the lithium.

In the meantime, I was trying to live my life, although not successfully. My students could tell that something was off. They never said anything to me, but I just couldn't be my best for them. I also started gaining weight very quickly. But Dr. Ashrot insisted that I stay on the lithium, so, mortifying as the weight gain was, I bought bigger clothing and kept moving. Still, I was totally distracted, and everything, even driving, was a nightmare. I started to ask Dr. Ashrot if he could put me back in the hospital to help me adjust my medication. But they had no beds.

One afternoon, I was driving north on the turnpike towards Hoboken. I was trying to make a left turn at a place where I remembered that there was a left turn option. It was not until I had initiated the turn at the green light that I realized that they had changed the intersection, and left turns were no longer allowed. I heard a loud smack, followed by a crash. My body jerked forward hard, and I felt instant shame and despair. I had driven right into the side of a Lexus.

This was not my first accident due to unfocused driving while feeling depressed. In the years I was really suffering, I got into about five car accidents. I'm not proud of this. I could have been killed or killed someone else by the way I was driving, but it was a symptom of my illness that I must accept.

The gold Lexus SUV and I pulled over to a local gas station. A very kind man got out. "Are you OK?" he said. I nodded and extended the same question to him.

"Yes, we're fine," he said. I hadn't realized until that point that there was a passenger in the car. I looked, and an elderly woman with curly plum-colored hair and wearing dark sunglasses was still sitting in the front passenger seat, shaking her head in disbelief.

The man looked at my car. I had a sticker on the back of it that read: "Columbia Alumni." He said, "You're Columbia?" to which I nodded. "I'm Dartmouth," he said proudly.

At that moment, it didn't matter to me what schools we both went to. I was just grateful to be alive and that I hadn't killed anyone else. I started sobbing. At that point the elderly lady with the plum hair approached us. "Why are *you* crying? *I* should be crying. You're an idiot, and could have killed me!" I was too shaken up to answer her, and Dartmouth tried to calm her down. He had called the police, and they were just getting to the scene. I was still sobbing uncontrollably.

"What's wrong?" Dartmouth said.

"I'm supposed to be in the hospital right now; they just don't have a bed for me," I said.

What happened next was a flurry of sirens and police and reports, and frankly, I don't remember most of it. I just remember calling Dr. Ashrot and telling him what happened.

"Oh, shit," he said. "You need to be in the hospital, now. I'll make sure they have a bed."

I felt deeply ashamed to be back in the hospital after many years of being hospital-free. In many ways, it felt like a failure, and I felt doomed to go back to being institutionalized. The hospital unit that I was on was a quiet one, and it gave me some time to reflect. As I lay in my bed, I thought about teaching. I was starting to feel quite unhappy with my job and very stressed by it. My principal didn't like me, I was too depressed to be any good to the kids, and I was gaining weight by the minute.

I complained about the fact that I was gaining weight to Dr. Ashrot in the hospital, and he said, "I know you're blowing up. But I'm not taking you off the lithium."

Many people have the luxury of being unhappy. They can stay miserable with little consequence besides their own misery. For me, unhappiness can equal suicidal thoughts, which can eventually lead to suicidal actions. I just cannot afford to be unhappy.

I thought about this during my time in the dingy Bayonne psych hospital. I knew in my heart that I needed to make a change. After the hospital, I brushed myself off and went right back to teaching. My students were noticing my weight gain, and many of them asked me if I was pregnant, which I found mortifying and depressing in and of itself. I contemplated suicide all the time, but tried to move through it to finish the school year, which I did successfully.

One day, I received a letter in the mail. It was from Dr. Ashrot.

"Dear Ms. Grossman,

"Because of several no-shows, I am closing your case. I wish you the best in your future endeavors."

"What an asshole," I thought. I didn't remember any no-shows, and I'd never been closed by a doctor like that before, right when I was my most vulnerable. Now it was just me, the lithium, and fifty extra pounds making our way into summer of '08.

The next key to becoming your best self is learning to ride the waves of your emotions. You may be wondering how I was able to be having suicidal thoughts while working and living my life. My answer is this: I knew that they were just thoughts and feelings.

While I was deeply depressed during my second year of teaching, I knew something that I hadn't known initially about my struggles—that they always pass. Like waves in the ocean, they come and go. This is why, in order to function through tough times and get to the other side, you must learn to surf.

"Urge surfing" is a strategy that I came across doing some research on how to help my clients overcome addiction, but it can be used for any negative emotion. When most people feel negative emotions, their urge is to take action to get rid of them. When they feel angry, they yell or fight; when they feel anxious, they do something to get rid of the anxiety—some even drink, smoke, or engage in other toxic, addictive habits. This would be good if it worked. But usually acting on negative emotions makes things much worse. If you are angry at your boss and then you punch him, now you have two problems instead of one. This may seem like an extreme example, but the truth is, any time you act on an emotion, you end up with two problems instead of one.

Urge surfing is one of many antidotes to this problem. It helps you to tolerate your emotions without acting on them so that they can pass more quickly. Here's what you do: first lie down or sit in a comfortable position. Then notice in your body exactly where the negative emotion is caught. For me, I feel my negative emotions in my throat. When I'm in any way stressed, angry, or sad, my throat feels tight and sore. It feels as though I've swallowed a pill that didn't make it all the way down my esophagus and got stuck.

Notice this feeling, wherever it manifests. Next, take a long breath and direct that breath towards that area of your body. Then let it out. Try to keep your full concentration on the area of your body that's holding the emotion and continue to direct your breath towards it. Little by little, the emotion will start to dwindle.

Emotions don't want to be willed away, stuffed down with food or alcohol, or numbed by drugs. They want to be acknowledged, which is what urge surfing does. It's important not to fear your feelings, because if you do, they become larger and more powerful. The way out of fearing emotions is remembering that they pass. Try watching the clock next time you feel an intense emotion to see how long it actually lasts while you are urge surfing. You'll be surprised to notice that when you don't act on an emotion or jump-start it by rethinking the negative thoughts that got you there to begin with, the emotion can pass in minutes.

This is how it was for me with suicidal thoughts and the sadness that accompanied them. I would have them, sometimes even daily, but if I continued through my day as if they weren't there and didn't get too unnerved by them, the sadness would go away, and the thoughts would leave with the sadness. And so I learned to function despite symptoms such as suicidal thoughts, anxiety, depression, and even psychosis. As I've said, during the semester that I was trying to graduate college, I was quite psychotic. But I continued to go about my schoolwork and finish anyway. I didn't give my thoughts and delusions power, and eventually they went away.

Whether urge surfing is the right technique for you or not, the key is to find some way to tolerate negative emotions and thoughts, without acting on them, until they pass. Remember, you are in charge of your emotions; your emotions are not in charge of you.

My next year of teaching, which began in the fall of 2008, was pretty much a disaster. I had now gained over 100 pounds, and my once slender 116-pound body was enormous. This fact alone created even more intense thoughts about suicide. I couldn't be there for the kids as I had been in the past. I tried really hard, but I just couldn't make it work. Also, I still wanted to make a difference in mental health.

I began researching ways that I could do this. I considered all kinds of graduate programs in mental health, but they were all so expensive, and remember, I was $60,000 in debt from Columbia. I didn't want to take out yet another student loan. I began to chant about my future. When I am depressed, I really struggle to chant, so I had fallen off from doing it for a while, even though I really needed it. I sat down in earnest one night and chanted for a way to accomplish my dreams.

The next day, I was doing more research, and I found a free program called Consumer Connections, which trained people with experience in the mental health system to be "peer providers." A peer provider is someone with lived experience of mental illness who helps others to recover from their struggles. It was the perfect fit for me, and I knew it right away. The one problem was, the next training course started in April, and it took place during the day.

In the meantime, things at school got so bad that I decided, in my tenure year, to resign. I knew at that point that teaching in a public school was just not working, and I was extremely miserable doing it. I agreed to work out the rest of my contract for the sake of my students.

I remember my conversation with the union representative at school when I shared my resignation with him. Paul was one of the band directors in addition to being one of the school's union leaders. Our conversation went something like this:

"Paul, I'm giving my resignation. I will work the rest of the year, but after that, I am choosing not to come back to school for the fall," I said, my lip quivering. I refused to cry in front of him.

"Emily," Paul said, "are you out of your mind? You are in your tenure year, and you have a stable job *with a pension* while the economy is awful. I can't imagine why you would leave. Aren't you terrified? What are you going to do instead?"

"I don't know yet, Paul, I just know it can't be this. It's not good for me, and it's not good for my students," I said, refusing to show my fear.

I knew that I had the rest of the school year to figure things out. I really wanted to go to Consumer Connections and get a job as a peer provider, but I didn't know how that would happen.

Although I didn't have any ideas, the Universe did. I continued to chant, attempting to try to manifest this sharp turn in my career. I felt awful—sick and sluggish and very sad. By that point, I had outed myself to Mrs. Worthington about being bipolar, and I think she took pity on me, because I started to see a much softer side of her: she was fighting for me.

Yet my suicidal thoughts were getting so bad that I couldn't be in school, and Mrs. Worthington knew it. One day she called me and told me that they had found a replacement for me, and I was not to continue the rest of the school year. I was crushed, but I knew that she made the right call. I chanted and asked the superintendent to pay me for the rest of my contract, and I'm grateful that he and the school board agreed to do this.

Sad as I was, this happened in late March, meaning that I could go to Consumer Connections, and I would be paid to do it! The Universe had closed a door with a gentle nudge, but a huge window had indeed opened at the same time.

The next key to being your best self is to be authentic. Authenticity is being your true self without being afraid. American society is always telling us to improve ourselves, giving us the subtle message that we are not OK as we are. We see commercials trying to sell us everything from the next hot car to a new hot body—all with the messaging that until we drive said car or have said body, we will not be good enough. The irony is that to be the best person that you can be, and to bring your unique gifts and talents to the world, you need to be comfortable with who and what you are. There is something that you can do better than anyone else. The key to figuring out what that is and bringing it to the world is to be who you really are.

I hope that you can see from this chapter that while teaching in a public school, I couldn't be my authentic self. I didn't tell my administration until the very end that I had bipolar disorder, because I feared that I would lose my job. I was also afraid that if my students' parents knew, they would not want me to teach their children. So I had to hide a very important part of who I was.

Additionally, my soul wanted something different. I knew that my true mission should be to find a way to help people suffering from mental illnesses. I saw this as more and more students came to me with their own mental health struggles. As I've said, as a teacher, I was powerless to truly help them.

So how do you know when you are being your authentic self? Let's start with how you know when you are *not* being your authentic self. The way I know when I am off the path of my authentic self is when I am struggling to get things done. It feels as if the force of the entire Universe is working against me. I'm trying to make it work, but it's as if I'm trying to squeeze something the size of a grapefruit out of something the size of a lime. It just doesn't fit.

Conversely, when I am being my authentic self, I feel whole and energized. Work is not an effort; I'm buzzing with enthusiasm and excited to begin each day. I feel I'm giving the best to the world, because I am. I notice that when I'm involved in tasks and I'm being my authentic self, time passes extremely quickly. I also notice that I am kinder to others, because Spirit is working through me and with me. I'm not struggling against anything, especially not myself. I feel as if I could reach up and ingest the moon, although really it and the rest of the Universe are temporarily ingesting me. I feel one with everything and nearly everyone.

There is a stark contrast between who I am when I am commuting to work from Montclair, New Jersey, to New York City every day and who I am at other times. My authentic self doesn't fit in well with the other commuters. Many of them are impatient and nasty. Many commute into the city to do purposeless jobs that make them a ton of money but crush their souls. When I am riding on the train, I'm in defense mode. I am trying to protect myself from the negativity of the people around me and preserve my energy for the workday. So I'm not always connected with the Higher Intelligence. I'm not as nice to people as I would like to be. Sometimes I become impatient and even angry. I'm not a train commuter by nature. I much prefer walking or driving. Yet public transportation is the only way for me to get to my job, so I tolerate an inauthentic situation.

Conversely, when I get to work, I'm usually quite joyful. My job is truly authentic to who I am as a human being. I feel connected with my colleagues and boss. I feel whole and complete. I feel grateful and free on most days. And I am highly productive. My job is a source of comfort during difficult times. Last year, I had a big family crisis, and every day was quite difficult. Yet at work, I could put it all aside, get things done, and feel like myself.

I also know that writing this book is authentic. I am writing it quickly, as if the words are pouring out of me. That's because they are. I feel called to write this book so that I can help others. I feel that all parts of me are present when I am writing. This is how I know that I am on the correct path.

I think back to when I was studying Michelangelo in school. I remember my teacher telling us that when Michelangelo was carving his statue of David out of marble, he felt as though David was already in the stone, and he just had to remove the other parts to get to him.

This was only true for Michelangelo because carving statues was a part of his authentic self. If I tried to carve a statue, it would end up looking like a block of Swiss cheese, because being a sculptor is not my mission, and I'm not my authentic self while doing it; I'm my frustrated self.

In *The Seven Spiritual Laws of Success*, Deepak Chopra talks about how our bodies indicate whether we are on the correct, authentic path even before we make a choice. He says that when we are about to make a positive choice for ourselves, we can really feel an energy flow through us, but we have a blocked feeling when we are about to make a choice that is not in line with our true selves.

The energy that I feel when I am on my path involves a tingling sensation. My feet tingle, my heart feels very light in my chest, and my throat loosens. When I am not on my path, the energy feels quite heavy. It's as if a truck just parked on my chest. My throat tightens, and I feel as if a lump of coal is stuck in it.

These are just some clues about being authentic. I encourage you to experiment with this. I believe that even small choices can be authentic or inauthentic. Choices such as "Do I drink water or orange juice today?" can be in line with your Highest Good or out of line with it. The next time you have a simple choice like this to make, try to see what happens if you get quiet and truly listen to your body before making a choice. You will probably feel something, even if it's subtle. If it's an important choice, you will feel it more strongly.

I encourage you to get on the path towards your authentic self so that you can know the happiness, peace, and serenity that I know today. It may take time for you to find yourself, but I guarantee that it is well worth the journey.

Turn Poison into Medicine

When I walked into the training room for Consumer Connections in the spring of 2009, I instantly felt at home. There were a few other people in the room, which was set up classroom style, with a PowerPoint projected on a screen in the middle of the room. I started to study the other people. They were all dressed casually and were sitting with eager anticipation. I felt a kinship to each of them without even speaking with them. These were my people; people who had walked a path like mine with their mental health and had gotten to the other side of it. I was proud to be in this room, because I knew it contained the fighters: the people who would not be stopped by something even as tragic as a mental illness.

I took a seat right in front. I was always nerdy like this, and at this stage of my life, I felt kind of proud of that. In a few minutes, a man whom I presumed to be our trainer walked in. He had great energy right from the start. He was a tall African-American man with a bald head, which shone like a halo over his scalp. He was dressed in a purple checked button-down shirt and black slacks, with square-tipped black leather shoes.

He saw me sitting in the front of the room and said, "Hi! I'm Frank Garris, and I'm going to be your trainer."

"Hi," I said, trying to mirror his warmth with my own. "I'm Emily, and I'm really happy to be here."

Frank smiled and went to the center of the room. It was time to start the class. There were about twelve of us at this point, and we had all had to apply to get there. I felt honored to be among the people chosen, as I had no previous work history in mental health.

"Hello, all," Frank said energetically to the class. "I'm Frank Garris, and I am going to be training you all to become peer specialists. After finishing this course, you will not only be able to get a job in the mental health field by using your own lived experience, you will also, after having work hours, be able to receive your New Jersey State Peer Specialist Certification."

My face lit up. This was thrilling to me. I knew that I had a mission in mental health, and the idea that I could get a job in the mental health field where my experiences coming to recovery were the main credential was exciting. I wondered why this program hadn't been developed decades ago. It made so much sense: the best person to encourage a person to recover is someone living in recovery themselves.

A side note here: When I entered the program, I was coming off a very shaky period with my own mental health. I recommend that people live in recovery for some time before trying to become mental health providers themselves. That said, recovery does not mean cure. There is no known cure for mental illness. Yet people can live highly productive, happy, healthy lives even if they have a mental illness. This is what I mean by recovery. I believe that everyone defines their own recovery. There comes a point where a person knows inside that they are living in recovery. This does not mean that there are no bumps.

I do not view my previous struggle teaching as a full relapse. I continued to function to the best of my ability and only wound up in the hospital for a short time. I still believe that I was living a recovered life at that time. I was living independently, I was doing my best to find meaningful work, and I was taking care of my responsibilities.

To get back to the Consumer Connections course, it consisted of six weeks of training, three times a week, for seven hours a day. During this time, Frank and a few other trainers taught us the basics. We learned about medications, diagnoses, Social Security and other entitlements, and we also learned some extremely valuable counseling skills. My favorite part was the role plays. I volunteered often, because I really wanted to practice and hone my skills. I found that counseling in this role came quite naturally to me.

I was also determined to get a job right away. I applied on my off time to every mental health agency that I could find. But the course was winding down, and I still hadn't heard from any of them. I found the number for human resources at one agency that I wanted to work in which was quite close to my apartment. I took a deep breath and dialed the number.

"Hello?" said a voice on the other end of the phone.

"Hi," I replied, trying to sound my most confident and professional. "My name is Emily Grossman, and I had applied online for the peer specialist position listed on your website, and I just wanted to confirm that you received my résumé."

"No, I haven't," the woman said, a bit perplexed. "Let me look in our system." She put me on hold to take a minute to look, and soon she was back on the line. "Ms. Grossman, yes, I have your résumé right in front of me. We'd love to have you in for an interview. When can you come in?"

"I'm free tomorrow," I said, trying not to sound overly eager. Inside, I was quite excited.

"Sure," the HR woman said. "Please be here at one o'clock tomorrow."

I felt a buzz of excitement. I barely slept that night. I knew that a good change was on its way.

The interview went smoothly. The program, called Crossroads to Wellness, sounded cool. It was in a community mental health center and was an outpatient program, meaning that clients did not stay there overnight. The program's objective was to get people right as they were coming out of the hospital and work with them for a short amount of time while they waited for longer-term care. They typically saw clients for three to five months. The waiting time for community mental health treatment on an outpatient basis was usually this long, so they would follow the person while they were on the waiting list until they could receive the proper care. I chanted fiercely that I would get the job.

I heard from Nancy, the program director, the next day. She offered me the job, which I accepted. I would take a $10,000 pay cut from my already meager teacher's salary, but I knew that it was worth it, and I chanted that somehow the Greater Good would make it up to me, and that I could live more frugally. I was still being paid by the board of education, so at least for a few months, I could collect two salaries. In addition, my father suggested that I cash in my pension, which I did, giving me another $5,000 in the bank to work with. That said, I was not very good with money; I was only able to make it work because of ramen noodles and my parents' financial help. For this, I am eternally grateful.

At Crossroads to Wellness, I worked on a team that was supervised by a psychiatrist and consisted of two social workers, a psychiatric nurse practitioner, and a social worker that specialized in working with the Korean population, which was very large in that area. I loved the work. I would sit in on all the clinical meetings, so I learned how to present cases, how diagnoses were decided upon, and what forms of treatment were appropriate for people with a variety of different diagnoses. I also worked with clients one-on-one, teaching them coping strategies, counseling them about their careers and going back to school. I also got to design curricula for groups and run them. I loved this. Finally I was teaching a subject that I believed in—giving people the tools and skills to recover from mental illness.

We worked with people of every race, illness, socioeconomic status, and religion. We worked with people in the criminal justice system. We fought hard for our clients and got to see some great successes. I was proud of the work that I was doing, and I learned very much from this opportunity. But the best part was that I was using my struggles to help others—something that I had always dreamed of doing.

* * *

Another important key to becoming your Highest Self is learning how to turn poison into medicine. This is an expression that we say in the Soka Gakkai all the time. It means that when you struggle with something in your life, you can turn it around for the Highest Good. It's another way of saying the popular expression "turning lemons into lemonade."

My perceived "poison" was obviously my mental health challenges. For many years, I felt I was being pulled into a deep abyss with no way out. I couldn't imagine how to turn my life around. But I knew something from a young age: I wanted to make a difference in other people's lives. I just didn't know how; nor did I believe that I had a skill set for doing this.

Finding Consumer Connections and learning that I could use my negative experiences to help others certainly turned poison into medicine for me. It made me feel as though all my struggles had happened for an important reason—to help me to serve others. I felt, and still feel, that my path had value because I could help other people through something similar. How empowering!

The next time you experience a poisonous situation in your life (which you inevitably will), I challenge you to work on turning it into medicine.

I have a friend from college whose young son struggles with a rare disease. He has been in the hospital many times and has had several operations. My friend has been devoted to working hard to help her son; she has also put together a charity to raise money to help find a cure for this disease. She and her husband encourage people to donate while they run marathons, and they also encourage others to join in. Because of this, their son's life has a meaning and a purpose that reaches far beyond just him.

My friend could have become very depressed when she found out about her son's condition. Instead, she and her husband chose to fight. She says, "We'll give anything but up." This is the attitude of people who are reaching for their Highest Selves. This is turning poison into medicine.

When we turn poison into medicine, we inevitably come face-to-face with at least part of our purpose on this earth. I believe it is my mission to heal others with my story. I couldn't do that if I didn't have a story to tell.

What is your greatest challenge in life? What is *your* poison? I challenge you to see how you can use it to benefit others. It's not just for them; it's for you as well. Using a challenge to serve others takes you out of your head, out of your own ego. And ego is where all the problems lie.

Turning poison into medicine has been the foundation of many important organizations. The first one that comes to mind for me is the Twelve Step fellowships. Their purpose is to help people who are struggling with addiction. In order to overcome an addiction like alcoholism, one is encouraged to serve others by "sponsoring" them and helping them to stay clean and sober. A popular saying in Alcoholics Anonymous is, "You cannot keep it unless you give it away"—meaning that you cannot maintain sobriety without working with another alcoholic and helping them to recover. This is a perfect example of turning poison into medicine.

My mother has a saying: "None of us get through this life unscathed." We all have problems, and at some point in everyone's life a problem will come down the pike that seems insurmountable.

That is when you have a choice. You can cross your arms and say, "This is not the script I ordered for the movie that is my life" and ruminate about how bad you have it. This will inevitably solve nothing and keep you stuck. The other option is to turn poison into medicine. Take it from me—it's much more fulfilling and healing to do this. Who knows? You just might change the world in the process.

Practice Self-Care

In the spring of 2010, during my time at Crossroads to Wellness, I began to have some symptoms again. I was very depressed because I was still not able to take off the hundred pounds that I had gained when Dr. Ashrot prescribed lithium, although he had long ago taken me off of it. I was also struggling a bit interpersonally on the job because I was depressed and feeling irritable. I realized that I would need to seek treatment again. However, I really wanted to make sure that I got the correct help.

I did a bit of research and found out that the best place where I could go for a refresher on dialectical behavior therapy (DBT) was in Connecticut. I didn't need to go inpatient, but I did need the support, and they had an intensive outpatient program that looked like a good fit.

I was nervous that I would lose my job, but I also knew that if I didn't go, I would either lose my job or just end up in another inpatient hospital. Mental illness can be like this—one often has to make difficult choices in order to take care of oneself. I sat down with HR, and through the Family Medical Leave Act (FMLA), I would still be paid a certain percentage of my salary for the weeks I was gone. The program was a four-week-long intensive program. I decided that I would go and commute up to Connecticut and back to New Jersey every day.

The program was on the grounds of Silver Hill Hospital in New Canaan, which is a beautiful place. Since it's a private hospital, there are enough funds to manicure the rolling hills and put red flowers in flower boxes on the windows. People can stay there as inpatients and then "graduate" to apartment-style houses. I was very grateful that my insurance covered Silver Hill, because on my own I would have never been able to afford it.

I walked into the room where our group would be held, eager to brush up my skills and learn some new ones. But as I looked around the beige and powder blue room, I couldn't help but feel a bit guilty. Was I doing the right thing by taking time off? Would I have a job when I returned? It felt like such a luxury to be at Silver Hill, but I knew in my heart that it was a necessity.

The group leader walked into the room and interrupted my thinking. "Hi everyone, my name is Linda. Welcome to group," she said. Linda had blazing red hair and a fiery disposition to match. I was hoping desperately that this group would be as good as the one Sherrie had run.

"Everyone, take your seats," Linda continued. "It's time to start." Behind Linda was a whiteboard, which she began to write on. "Today we are going to do mindfulness," she continued. "Who remembers what that skill is?"

Always eager to be teacher's pet, I raised my hand. There was a comfort in how familiar this all was, and I really wanted to make the skills my own this time.

"Mindfulness," I said, "is being in the moment." I sat back with great confidence that I had answered correctly and noticed a few of the other people in the group eyeing me with annoyance. No one likes a teacher's pet.

One guy in the group was really attractive, but I knew that it was not good to date people in the group. We all had our own issues to work through, and the worst thing that could happen to me was to have a difficult relationship when I was so vulnerable. Besides, at 220 pounds, I wasn't feeling attractive anyway.

Linda looked at me. "Emily," she said, "is that your name?" I nodded. "Well, Emily, what you said is accurate, but mindfulness goes deeper than that. Mindfulness is the ultimate act of self-care."

Whoa. There was that word again. I had heard it in many of my groups, but I had no idea how to practice it or how it related to mindfulness.

As if reading my mind, Linda went on. "Think about it, everyone. Mindfulness is keeping your mind in the here and now. And right now nothing is wrong. We are just sitting in a room, having a conversation about mindfulness. Yet most of you are probably not fully here with your minds. You are either thinking about your past with regret or thinking about your future with anxiety. The best way to care for yourself is to take care of your thoughts. And the best way to take care of your thoughts is to keep them in the present, because that is where the peace is—it's right in the here and now."

Wow! She was so right. I knew that I spent a large percentage of my life beating myself up about my illness and all the years that I had "lost" trying to recover. When I wasn't doing that, my mind's other favorite channel was the one that told me to be anxious about my career and the way it would evolve. I had never thought that this was not practicing self-care.

The next key to becoming your Highest Self is self-care. I used to think that self-care involved getting my hair and nails done or getting a massage. While those things can be a part of self-care if you enjoy them (I personally don't like massages), as I found out in my DBT class, self-care goes way deeper than this.

The kind of self-care that I'm talking about involves many things, including such a deep love for yourself that you are willing to do anything to protect and care for yourself. There are many ways I practice self-care, and I'll tell you about some of them now. Please bear in mind, though, that we will only be scratching the surface.

The first thing that I'm very strict about is having structure to my day. This is self-care for my mind, because when I have too much downtime, I'm vulnerable to getting stuck in fear and anxiety and losing forward motion. So I try to fill even my days off with meaningful activities and events. I make plans with friends, I get my errands done, and I schedule some time to rest as well.

Chanting is another thing that I try to do every day for self-care. When I chant, I can be more present for the rest of the day. I also use chanting to get answers through intuition to my life's most pressing problems. It helps me to manifest my desires, as long as they are in line with the Highest Good. Most importantly, chanting is my way of connecting with my Higher Power.

I try to exercise as regularly as possible. My body isn't able to do the kind of high-impact cardio that it once could, but I do try to walk regularly and lift weights. I know that as I continue to lose weight and improve my fitness, all of this will change.

Speaking of weight loss—I identified about seven months ago that this had to be a priority. At five feet three and 220 pounds, I was not able to function at an optimal level. I joined a Twelve Step program. Actually I had been going on and off to this program for compulsive overeaters and food addicts for years. But until seven months ago, it hadn't stuck.

Yet seven months ago, I made a decision: if I was going to talk to people about how I had become my best self, I couldn't be well over 200 pounds. If I was going to live a healthy life, it had to be mind, spirit, and *body*, not just mind and spirit.

I am blessed to have met my current sponsor in this program. She, like me, had been in and out of the program for many years without getting better. She is smart, reliable, dedicated, and most of all, knows my disease of food addiction inside out. She is a true teacher and mentor. I've been working my butt off with her spiritually and physically to overcome my eating disorder once and for all (and I've so far lost sixty-nine pounds).

I do several different things daily to maintain my recovery from food addiction. I read literature from the program and write about it every day. I call my sponsor and three other people from the program every day as well. I report my food to my sponsor before I take a bite, and my food is free of sugar, flour, wheat, caffeine, alcohol, and artificial sweetener. I weigh and measure everything. I attend meetings during the week. That's my physical self-care.

Another important aspect of self-care for me is having boundaries. I have found that because I'm a people pleaser by nature, I want to say yes to every request I get. But I've learned the hard way that when I do that, I get burnt out. So I've started saying no to people and letting them know what my limits are around work and play. If I'm too tired and someone asks me to make plans, I schedule for another day. If someone asks me to give them advice on mental health, I tell them that I'm happy to, but I explain that because I do this for a living, I do have to charge for my services. These things are awkward at times, but they protect me and my time, and I've become much calmer and less overwhelmed as a result.

I am also learning to take care of my responsibilities and not let things pile up. This is an important aspect of self-care as well. I used to have a messy apartment most of the time. I was disorganized with things like bill paying, getting my oil changed on my car, and many other things. I realized that when I do the laundry and shop for food regularly, I'm actually taking care of myself. I am loving myself just as my own mother loves me, as these are all things that she once did for me.

A final aspect of self-care that I've gotten better about is going to doctors. I used to avoid getting regular check-ups because I was afraid to get bad news. Also, who likes to sit naked in front of a near stranger as they inspect the most intimate parts of your body? But I've learned to stay on top of these things because I want to live a long and healthy life and inspire others—something that I cannot do if I'm sick.

Self-care is not selfish. It's the ultimate act of self-love and an important portal towards your Higher Self. We were meant to love and care for ourselves. People who spend their lives overly sacrificing for others or beating themselves up for every kind act that they do for themselves do not become their best selves.

Conversely, when you take authentic steps to love and care for yourself, it's amazing what starts to happen. This is when true peace begins to set in. It's a gorgeous experience that I hope you will have after learning to care for yourself.

Find Happiness Within

I returned from the DBT group feeling slightly better, but not fully back to my old self. I hadn't made a dent in weight loss, and this was stressing me out. It was getting to the point where I was associating certain locations with the foods I would eat there.

"Oh," I would think, "at the Starbucks on Route 46, there are delicious brownies. Exit 142 off of the Garden State Parkway has a Kentucky Fried Chicken, where I can stop and get a fast dinner." I knew that this was not good, but I didn't know what to do about it.

I tried almost everything from Weight Watchers to hypnosis to doctor-supervised meal plans. Nothing worked. I just couldn't overcome my weight, and I was feeling hopeless about it.

I remember the first Twelve Step meeting that I attended for my food addiction. It was around the time that I was at

Crossroads to Wellness in the summer of 2010. I had met my first sponsor on a phone meeting. She asked me to attend a meeting in Mount Kisco, New York, about an hour and a half from my home. I was desperate, so I went.

When I walked into the church where the meeting was held, I was immediately greeted by an attractive, blond-haired man with a warm smile. I was perplexed, because he was very thin, and because I was at a meeting for food addiction, I had assumed that everyone would be overweight like me. I felt my self-consciousness overcome me right away and started to blush.

"I'm Chris," the thin blond man said. "Are you new to the meeting?"

"Yes, I'm Emily," I said looking around. The room was like a school auditorium. There was a stage at the back end, covered by a large red velvet curtain. On the other end was a table set up with coffee and creamer. The walls had signs on them that said things like, "Easy does it," and one had the Twelve Steps.

I sat in one of the metal folding chairs that had been put in a circle. Because it was summer and the room was not air-conditioned, I felt my leg get stuck to the chair. This was a point of shame for me. I knew when I got up, you would be able to see the spots of sweat. Because I was so overweight, I sweated all the time, which was exacerbated by a room without air conditioning.

The blond man was now hugging a few women (also thin) who had just arrived. I felt more and more self-conscious about my size. Yet I was hoping that this would be it—that I would finally get the help I needed.

The meeting began shortly after. A woman read the Twelve Steps, which originated with Alcoholics Anonymous. The only difference was that she replaced the word "food" for the word "alcohol" and the words "compulsive overeater" for the word "alcoholic."

After this, we began reading from the Alcoholics Anonymous bible known as the Big Book. Written by an alcoholic named Bill W. back in the 1940s, it talked about his journey to sobriety and other people's journeys as well. It also gave instructions for overcoming addiction.

After each paragraph was read, someone would share from their own experience how it applied to them. I was amazed. In that room, I heard things about food and food addiction that I had never heard before.

The biggest thing that made an impression on me was when one woman said that she was eating to fill a "God-sized hole" inside of her. By this, she meant that she was using food to fill a void that only a Higher Power could fill.

These words rang so true to me. There I was, living in recovery from bipolar disorder, but I was far from happy. I was eating and stuffing down every negative emotion that I had. Was I too eating to fill a God-sized hole? I was sure that this was the case.

It reminded me very much of something that we say in Buddhism. We often talk about how if you are looking to something outside of yourself to bring you happiness and peace, you are not practicing correctly.

I was looking to food, something external, to make me happy on the inside. I realized that before food, I had looked to many other things to make me happy. In my teens and early twenties, I had jumped from boyfriend to boyfriend. When I was younger than this, I looked to school achievements and accolades. All of this was based on ego and self, and all of it was looking outside of myself for happiness.

Finding happiness within is the next key to becoming one's Higher Self. You may be wondering how to find that happiness. In my experience, it comes from two things: the first is being connected to and comfortable with yourself. The second, which is related to the first, is being connected to a Higher Power.

Let me talk about the first one first. When I was looking outside of myself for happiness, I was always expecting other people, places, and things to make me happy. I've learned that this is not only impossible, it's also unfair to put those expectations on someone or something outside yourself.

I think about times when I've been truly happy. These can be times with others, but many times I'm all by myself, making myself happy. Whether it's through listening to music, dancing, reading, or writing, the happiness of being comfortable while alone with myself has been pure and true. And I don't have to rely on anyone else to feel it.

I've learned to like being alone with myself. I enjoy the company I keep most of the time. I find myself funny and entertaining. I'm not saying this to be egotistical. I think we should all be lucky enough to feel this way, and I wish it for all of you. This connection to oneself is true happiness.

The other way I feel this true state of happiness is by connecting to my Higher Power. I do this through chanting, but there are many other ways. When I chant, I feel a lightness of being. My mind calms down, and I feel a strong, peaceful feeling. I feel incredibly grateful when these moments happen, because I'm able to get out of my head and the day's problems and remember that I am connected to the Source at all times. The only thing I have to do is take the time to chant and connect. This is the beauty of finding happiness by connecting to All There Is—it is always available to us.

Key 21

Lift Someone Else Up

In 2010, while at Crossroads to Wellness, I had several successes. One that I remember vividly was Justine. Justine was a young woman of no more than twenty-five. When she came to Crossroads, she was being prescribed a high level of anxiety medications and sleeping pills just to function. She lived at home, was sleeping through the day, and was not working or going to school.

I began working with Justine, giving her some of the coping strategies that I had learned through our DBT group. Justine thrived with these strategies and started to come out of the fog of her depression and anxiety. She even went off her anti-anxiety medication. She wanted to work in fashion. While we were working together, she got a job at Bergdorf Goodman and applied to the Fashion Institute of Technology in New York City.

While it was great that this client of mine was able to do so well, it paled in comparison to how I felt about working with her.

This is when I discovered one of the most important lessons that I would ever learn: to become your Higher Self, you must be giving back and helping to lift other people up.

You don't have to be working in a helping profession to do this. Maybe it just means spending time with an elderly family member or babysitting for a friend's child. The key is doing something that gets you out of your own head about yourself.

Furthermore, you have to bring out your best self in order to lift someone else up. Think about it. Let's say that a friend gets into trouble at work and needs to talk it out with someone. In order to help this friend, you can't be cranky or not at your best. For the moments that you are helping your friend talk through the situation, you are (hopefully) compassionate and loving. This is your Higher Self.

The more you take the time to lift up another, the less likely you are to dwell in your own inner negativity. When you are in this state of positivity, I believe that the Universe recognizes it and gives you more positivity. So helping another also helps you.

As I've said previously, in the Twelve Step world, we have a saying: "You can't keep your recovery unless you give it away." You are not going to stay well unless you help others by giving them your knowledge and wisdom about your own recovery. Sponsoring people keeps it green for you—it helps you remember how hard it was in the beginning and what you need to do to stay recovered.

The same is true with my mental health recovery. Becoming a peer provider brought so much to my life because helping others to recover helped me to remember all of the skills that I use to recover. There is nothing to remind you of your own skills like helping someone else to learn them. Teaching someone else is the best way to show that you understand a skill and can help someone else apply it.

In Buddhism, we are constantly talking about lifting up others—not just helping them, but enabling them to become capable leaders themselves so that they in turn can help others. As a Buddhist leader, you are trained to always look for someone who will replace you as you grow and move up the leadership chain. This is essential to helping the organization grow.

I wish that the same could be said about corporate environments. A smart organization does work this way. If they want to expand, they need capable leaders on all levels. The only way to do this is to have upper management lift people up to replace them as they grow into bigger positions.

If you really want to grow and become your best self, lift someone else up. The positive benefit to you will be just as great as it is to them, and you will see that the incredible feeling of watching someone rise is a reward in and of itself.

I worked in community mental health until 2012. My recovery became very strong. The more time I had out of the hospital and working, the better I felt. I was learning how to make DBT and coping skills a part of my daily practice. This, combined with chanting, made the magic begin to happen.

I began to feel an itch to get back into the classroom. I knew that I didn't want to teach in a public school again, but I wanted to teach something that I was truly passionate about: that recovery was 100 percent possible for people with mental illness. I realized that it was my true mission to heal and inspire others with my own journey to recovery.

I chanted and took part in a lot of Buddhist activities at this time, but I also networked like crazy. Sure enough, within four months, a contact in my network sent me a job posting that fit that description. It would be working for an organization called the New York Association of Psychiatric Rehabil-itation Services (NYAPRS). They were looking for a trainer to go around to the five boroughs of New York City, as well as Long Island, and train mental health professionals on recov-ery. I couldn't believe my eyes! It was the exact next career move that I wanted to make. And sure enough, I got the job.

One of our major clients was a state psychiatric hospital on Long Island. I remember the first time I arrived. It looked like a combination of a prison and a ghost town. The land-scaping was overgrown and weedy, and each building looked eerily like the one before it. I had to go through quite a maze to find where I was supposed to be, and when I did, I realized that I had to get through a lot of security to get into the build-ing. "Good thing I brought my ID," I thought.

My task was going to be to teach these professionals, who had been working with the same clients in the hospital for many years (and in some cases, many decades), that recovery is possible.

I remember the first training very well. It was an unsur-prisingly small turnout. The training was entitled, "Looking through a Recovery Lens." In it, I shared my story, talked about the theory of recovery, and helped clinicians to learn how to implement it. The buzz about this training around the hospital was negative. Even the participants were skeptical. How could people who were so chronically ill ever recover?

I was undeterred. I began: "I know that you probably had certain assumptions about me when I walked in the room. I appear to be a professional. I'm dressed that way, and I hope that I act that way also. But what if I told you that a decade ago, I was in a similar position to many of your clients?"

A hush fell over the participants as I continued. Some sat very erectly in their chairs. Others were shaking their heads in disbelief. I had them, and I knew it. The training went extremely well, although there was a lot of pushback. It was hard for these professionals to understand that I was once about to be hospitalized in a similar place myself. But they stayed with me, and little by little, even the sourest clinician in the room came around.

I closed with the following, by my hero Dr. Patricia Deegan:

It is not our job to pass judgment on who will and will not recover from mental illness and the spirit breaking effects of poverty, stigma, dehumanization, degradation and learned helplessness. Rather, our job is to participate in a conspiracy of hope. It is our job to form a community of hope which surrounds people with psychiatric disabilities. It is our job to create rehabilitation environments that are charged with opportunities for self-improvement. It is our job to nurture our staff in their special vocations of hope. It is our job to ask people with psychiatric disabilities what it is they want and need in order to grow and then to provide them with good soil in which a new life can secure its roots and grow. *And then, finally, it is our job to wait patiently, to sit with, to watch with wonder, and to witness with reverence the unfolding of another person's life.* [My emphasis]

After the training, I went upstairs to Jennifer Gallihan's office. Jennifer was a hospital administrator who was in my corner. She knew that the hospital had limitations in helping clients to get better and move on to independent living, and she was hoping this would change.

"How'd it go?" Jennifer said, twirling her honey-brown hair with a French manicured finger. Jennifer's office had those pale blue cinderblock walls, but she had warmed it up with colorful posters and pictures of her family.

"Well," I said, "they seemed responsive, but there were only four of them."

"That doesn't surprise me," Jennifer said, still twirling. "The hospital staff has been all abuzz since we talked about the idea of your training, but not in a good way. They just don't believe that recovery is possible, and they don't want to let anyone tell them differently."

"That doesn't surprise me either," I said, "but give me a few more months with them. I think we will see a change in attitudes."

"OK," Jennifer said with a skeptical tone.

My determination did not wane a bit. I knew that if I could get more of the staff in the room, I could change attitudes. It was just a matter of word spreading.

The next time I did training, I was running five minutes late. I hated being late, but the traffic on the Long Island Expressway had been terrible, and it was beyond my control. I comforted myself by knowing that it was going to probably be a small group.

When I walked into the room, I nearly fell down. There were about thirty mental health professionals waiting to be trained on recovery. Word had spread quicker than I had imagined possible.

It wasn't a fairy-tale turnaround. Many of the staff were quite skeptical. One psychiatrist in the room said, "If you look up the word *recovery* in the dictionary, you will see that it means *cure*. You can't cure people of mental illness."

"True," I said, "but you can help people to live a highly productive and stable life, get them back to living in the community, and help them work towards goals such as a job or school. In many cases, symptoms are reduced as a result."

He was not having it. In fact, he got up and left the training shortly thereafter. I tried not to be too hurt. I knew that it wasn't me: it was the material that I was presenting. I knew that I had to get the trust of the people in the room. I had an idea. After the break, I made a passionate plea to whoever was left in the room.

"Look," I said, "we all got into this field to help people, and I know that you are all doing wonderful work with the people that you serve. However, believing that people can recover makes your work easier. If you give clients choices and freedom to run their recovery the way they choose, you won't have to work so hard, because they will be on board with their goals, and they will do most of the work for you."

People's faces went from stern to soft to smiling and bright. I realized that these people weren't angry with me or my ideas. They were burned out from working in a backwards system. I was there to share the idea that if they worked smarter, their jobs could be easier and less stressful. The energy in the room lightened, and people got up to thank me.

I went back to Jennifer's office. "I think we're making a dent!" I said with enthusiasm.

"Excellent," Jennifer said. "I'm on your team. Keep up the great work."

The trainings continued to grow after this until I found myself presenting in an auditorium to hundreds. I succeeded because I had learned not to dismiss my haters or hate them back; I learned how to find what motivated them and use it to my advantage. I had learned how to turn enemies into friends.

This is a skill that I will pass on to you: If you want to be your best self, you need to avoid being discouraged by the haters. Instead, try to figure out how you can make their lives a bit easier, and be the person to help them. There is a saying that you catch more flies with honey than with vinegar. If you are kind and, more importantly, if you can bring value to your enemies, they will soon turn into friends.

Why is this so important to your well-being? When someone hates you, the impulse is to hate them right back, but this energy blocks you from the sunlight of the Spirit. It prevents you from connecting with your Higher Power. And we need that connection as much as possible to be our Higher Selves.

So the next time someone hates, remember what I've said. Look for a way to make their life sweeter. Chances are your life will become sweeter as well.

⸻𝄐 Key 23

Practice Compassion

In 2014, after working for two years at NYAPRS, another amazing opportunity came my way. It was working at Columbia Psychiatry, a clinic in New York City, where I would be a part of training teams all over the country to help youth with first episode psychosis to recover. The model was completely in line with my values, and I would still be training. I was hired soon thereafter.

The program, called OnTrackNY, was a cutting-edge treatment for youth experiencing psychosis: seeing and hearing things that weren't there. I loved the work, which involved some travel in the beginning. One of the first places that my colleagues and I visited was a large mental health center in Syracuse.

Aside from me, the entire team had their flights canceled because of inclement weather, and I was the only one to arrive. I realized immediately that I would be making the first impression on the mental health center. I would be representing the entire team.

When I first arrived, the executive director of the organization was waiting there for me. David was a tall, warm man, wearing a gray suit.

"Hi, Emily," he said in a kind way. "We're glad that you made it here safely. I have to say that we are a little disappointed that the rest of your team won't be joining us in person. We were looking forward to meeting everyone."

I knew that I had to act fast and compassionately. It wasn't our fault that the weather was bad and the rest of the team could not make it to Syracuse. Still, rather than being annoyed by David's comment, I tried to look at things from his perspective. It *was* a shame that our whole team couldn't make it to the training site. As a result, we would be doing most of the training remotely, and this is never the same as doing it in person.

"David, I'm so sorry that my team is not here. I know that this must really be disappointing for you and your team. I promise that I will give my all to make sure that the training exceeds your expectations."

David immediately softened. "Thank you, Emily. We look forward to the training." It was a wonderful success, and David became one of my biggest supporters.

What worked so well? I put myself in David's shoes, which is another way of saying that I practiced compassion. I had to look at the situation from his perspective and validate his frustrations. After all, he and his team were our customers.

* * *

Compassion is an important skill to master on the journey to becoming your Higher Self. When we can learn to look at other people's viewpoints instead of clinging strongly to our own, our hearts soften, and we become more able to forge deep, lasting relationships. And relationships are very important to becoming our Higher Self.

But it's not just important to have compassion for others; it is important to have for yourself as well. Mental illness is very challenging. It can sabotage relationships and destroy one's dreams, albeit temporarily. One thing I had to learn when these things happened was to have compassion for myself.

Recently my therapist described self-compassion and self-love as picturing a loving mother that is inside of you at all times. This mother figure doesn't judge you or treat you harshly. She loves you without conditions. Self-compassion is truly about loving yourself, no matter what.

How do you do this? While I'm still learning this lesson, I can say that self-talk is a large part of it. It is important to say nice things to yourself. I know that this is basic advice, but how often do you do it? How often do you catch yourself speaking unkindly to yourself?

The key to self-love is "acting as if." Even if you don't believe the kind things that you are saying to yourself at first, keep going! If you hear these kind words often enough, eventually your brain will believe them.

I also use mantras. When I feel a negative thought about myself coming up, I say, "I love myself, and I love my life" over and over again until the negative thought goes away. I even have trained myself to say this as I walk through the streets of New York City to and from work. Little by little, I have started to believe these thoughts. And the truth is, I do love myself and my life!

The more I have been able to practice compassion for others and myself, the better I've felt. As I've explained in earlier chapters, being angry at others is a luxury that people cannot afford if they want to be their Higher Selves. Anger blocks us off from our connection, and we cannot be our Higher Self if we are not connected to our Higher Power. Self-compassion and self-love are also critical. If you are busy being angry at yourself all the time, you cannot overcome negativity and shine as your best self.

Remember—you were created by Love with love. You deserve to love others and yourself, and you cannot accomplish this without compassion.

Seek Guidance

I'm in my Buddhist center in New York City. It is the spring of 2017, and I decide to go after work to chant with others. I find that practicing with a group really strengthens my own practice. I climb up the pale pink marble stairs towards the second floor to do evening *gongyo*, which is chanting *nam myoho renge kyo*, but also the recitation of parts of the Lotus Sutra, which was one of the Buddha's final teachings. When I get to the second floor of the New York City Culture Center, I am greeted by two *byakuran*, or female ushers. They are wearing navy blue suits with white button-down shirts, and each has a yellow and blue scarf tied around her neck.

I sit down in a rust-colored cushioned folding chair and begin to chant. The people are chanting loudly and quickly, and I begin to absorb the harmonious sound, basking in it as if it were rays of the sun. The sound fills me up, and as I chant in front of the large gohonzon in the center of the room, the anxiety and stressors of the day melt like a snow cone.

It seems like only minutes have passed, but when I look at the clock, I realize it has been a half hour. A *gajokai*, one of the male ushers, rings the large golden U-shaped bell at the center of the room near the gohonzon. He is wearing black pants and a white button-down shirt with a red tie. He can't be more than twenty, but he looks so responsible up there. My heart fills with pride.

"Good evening," he says, "for tonight's daily activities, open chanting will be on the fifth floor, there is a chapter meeting on the third floor in room 302, an introductory meeting in room 303, and finally guidance in the library."

I grab my bag and race upstairs for guidance, hoping that I'll be the first one to the library. In Nichiren Buddhism, guidance is given by more experienced members who have been practicing for a significant length of time. They advise others on how to practice correctly and infuse Buddhism into their lives.

Sure enough, I'm first. "Yes!" I think, noting that it must be meant to be that I am up there at that time. Usually when there is alignment like that, I know that it means that I have something to learn from this person.

I walk into a room, and a woman that I've never met before is sitting at the large wooden table in the library. It is a square room with wooden bookshelves on three of its sides, and it is full of the writings of both our founder, Nichiren Daishonin, and our presidents, including Daisaku Ikeda.

The woman has short gray hair and dark brown eyes. I guess that she is my parents' age, although I can never be sure. "Have a seat," she says warmly. "My name is Natalie."

"Hi, Natalie," I say, trying to mirror her warmth, "I'm Emily."

"What would you like to talk about today?" Natalie asks sincerely, turning up her hearing aid, which is somehow controlled by her iPhone.

"I'd like to talk about relationships." I say. "I've been practicing for eleven years now, and when I first started chanting, the very first thing I chanted about was finding my soul mate, but it still hasn't happened."

"Hmm," she mutters, "well, you've come to the right place. "I chanted for twenty years before it happened for me," she says matter-of-factly.

"Really?" I say.

"Yes," she replies. "I was married for thirty-four years to my soul mate, and I loved him. Recently he passed away, though."

"I'm sorry for your loss," I say, feeling very sympathetic.

"I should be a puddle on the floor with all of the things that life has dealt me. My son has schizophrenia, and he's in jail," she says, looking down, "but you know what? I'm truly joyful at this exact moment in time."

I blink in disbelief. "Really?" I ask, not trying to sound too shocked. I don't want her to feel bad, but it does sound as if life has given her a couple of tough blows.

"Yes, and I even went on a first date the other day," she continues with a twinkle in her eye.

"Wow. How do maintain your optimism despite your struggles?"

"Well, I chant, I seek guidance, just like you are doing right now, and I study buddhism," she says.

"That's it?" I ask feeling disappointed.

"Let me tell you a story, Emily," Natalie says, looking right into my eyes. "When I was going through the court system with my son, I didn't know how to chant about the situation. I got guidance from another woman leader who said, chant for the best outcome for you, your son, and all the world; chant for the best outcome for the peace of the world."

In Nichiren Buddhism, we believe that world peace, which we call *kosen-rufu*, can only be accomplished when each individual in the world becomes truly happy. I know this, so what Natalie is saying makes a lot of sense.

"The outcome of the court case was obviously not what I wanted," Natalie says. "No one wants their child behind bars. But the judge looked me right in the eye when he was sentencing him, and said, 'I know that your son will be able to come through this and contribute to society.' My son had struggled for years with schizophrenia and would not get help. In jail, he is getting help, and his schizophrenia is improving. Even though it wasn't the outcome that I wanted, it is the outcome that is making him the most happy, because he's getting treatment. And this makes me happy. He is also practicing every day in jail, something that I could have never twisted his arm to do before. The point of the story is that when we chant, the Universe always gives us what we need to become truly happy—even if it's not what we think we need. Let me ask you something, Emily," she says.

I nod to indicate that she may.

"You say that you've been chanting for this for eleven years, yet you haven't been in the right relationship all that time. What have you learned in the process?"

"Well," I say, thinking for a moment, "when I broke up with my last boyfriend, I knew that I had become very dependent on him. I was waiting for someone to save me from bipolar disorder and thought that he could do it, but we both found that he couldn't. During this time as a single person, I've learned to take care of myself. I've been forced to. And I'm living in recovery now. I did that for myself."

"Wow!" Natalie replied. "Now I'm encouraged! So you see, Emily, that the gohonzon and your chanting have brought you what you've needed in this time. Were you to have a relationship before you knew that you could truly depend upon yourself, you would have become too needy all over again and probably driven the new guy away. Mature relationships are not about two people needing each other; they are about two whole individuals joining together to bring something greater to the world."

"Thank you, Natalie," I say, wishing I could talk to her all day. "I really appreciate your support. Have a great day!" With that, I leave.

The next key to attaining your best self is seeking guidance. By guidance, I mean getting advice from people who are living the way you want to live. This could be a spiritual mentor, as in my case, or a friend, relative, teacher, coach, or anyone else you admire. You don't even have to know them that well, as was the case with Natalie. I went to Natalie because I knew that she was senior to me in faith and had been practicing a long time.

Regardless of whom you choose, it's important to go in with an open mind. I didn't expect that when I approached

Natalie, I would hear a story about her son being in jail. If you told me this fact about her ahead of time, I might have had a bias, thinking she could not have been practicing correctly if something that awful happened to her. But as I heard more of her story, I was deeply encouraged by her spirit and her ability to find joy even through the most difficult situations, and I left very encouraged, feeling that if she can find joy, I can too.

People need guidance about different things at different times. Perhaps you are going through a struggle in your romantic life, as I was. Perhaps you need guidance about your finances. No topic should be off-limits. You will only have difficulty if you have a problem but keep it inside of you.

The poet John Donne wrote that "no man is an island." We all need the support of others to get through life. I guarantee that whatever situation you find yourself in, someone in the world has been through the same or similar and has insight and advice to offer. You don't have to walk alone through difficult things.

I consider guidance like a tune-up of my soul. Much like an instrument that needs to be tuned in order to play on key, I need to be tuned in order to live as my best self. When I fall off course, guidance is there to get me back on track. I believe that God puts people in our path to be God's voice. While we cannot talk directly to Spirit, we can hear Spirit's words through others. On the day that I visited Natalie, I knew that she was only a channel. She reminded me of who I was and pointed out what I needed to learn.

It's a funny thing about guidance. Sometimes it just comes to you without your even seeking it out. The other day, I was having lunch with a friend. I was lamenting the fact that I had made a costly relationship mistake in my past by choosing to be with the wrong person when I had a choice of two different men. I was saying that had I made the other choice, life would have been much different. At that moment, she looked me right in the eyes and said, "The other guy didn't have the lesson that you needed to learn at that time." I know that that was the Divine speaking to me through her. Life will teach us what we need to know, so get ready to listen.

Be the Change

It's three o'clock in the afternoon, and I'm sitting at my gray cubicle at work. The organization I'm working for, which is the largest health and human services agency in New York, has 3,000 employees, and I'm charged with training them on how to provide mental health care that is focused on hope and client recovery.

I am writing a proposal for a new training series for peer providers, toggling back and forth between my two screens as I do research on the topic. I have just completed training some staff using my own mental health recovery story. Just as I am putting a period on the last sentence of my proposal, a colleague who was in the training approaches my desk.

"Emily," she says pensively, "your training today really impacted me, especially your story. I want you to know that tonight, I'm going to take my mental health medication and do all of the things necessary to take care of myself. Thank you!"

She has never before told me that she even has a mental health diagnosis, and I can only feel honored. This is not an anomaly. Many times when I share my story, people come over to me in this way. But it gets me every single time. I'm so grateful to be able to do this work and empower other people to share their stories as well. It's the main reason that I do what I do.

A familiar quote, which has been attributed to Gandhi, says, "You must be the change you wish to see in this world." The change that I want more than any in this world is to see the eradication of mental health stigma in my lifetime. I dream that one day, it will be OK for people to talk just as openly about their mental health as they do about their physical health. It is my hope and prayer that one day telling your employer that you need to take a mental health day will really be alright and going into treatment for mental illness does not have to be something that people talk about in hushed tones to only their closest friends and relatives.

To this end, I try to live my mental illness recovery out loud. Besides this book, I share my story at every opportunity I get. I have written about mental health recovery for the Huffington Post. I have been written up in newspapers and magazines speaking about my mental health. I do it all not for my ego, or to ride the fame train. I do it to help people. If I want to see the eradication of stigma in my lifetime, I have to do my part by telling my story to everyone who will listen. It's not just my own personal agenda; it's my mission.

Telling my story has had its difficulties. I am single, and I date online from time to time. As soon as a man Googles my name, he can find out all types of things about my mental health and treatment that are very personal yet are part of the public domain. The same is true for new friends. But I look at it this way—people are going to eventually find out anyway, so letting them know who I am up front is a self-selecting process. Either you accept me for who I am and you stay in my life, or you don't. I refuse to hide or try to change who I am for anyone anymore.

Despite these difficulties, I still wouldn't have it any other way. I'm not a martyr. I have a wonderful life full of a meaningful career and great relationships. And I have a cause and a mission to fight for—something that I really believe in. This keeps me vital and vibrant nearly all of the time.

My advice if you are feeling lost in your life right now is to *be* the change yourself. Think of an injustice. Think of an issue that you want to contribute to. Think about your own legacy during your short time on this planet. Rather than thinking about what you can get from a career and from others, think about what you can give.

I have a sign hanging on my desk that was given to me by a dear colleague while I worked training mental health professionals at Columbia Psychiatry. It says:

> We are visitors on this planet. We are here for ninety or one hundred years at the very most. During that period, we must try to do something good, something useful with our lives. If you contribute to other people's happiness, you find the true goal, the true meaning of life.
>
> —*H.H. the Fourteenth Dalai Lama*

* * *

To me, being the change is just this: finding your own unique way to transform your corner of the Universe. It is asking yourself not just what will make you truly happy in life, but what will make others happy as well. What is the best use of your time and talents to contribute to the peace of our planet? When you figure this out, you own the Universe inside of yourself, and you can use that force to create deep fulfillment, happiness, and success.

In the end, discovering your Highest Self isn't about the self at all. It's about being a conduit to your Higher Power to do that entity's good work. It's becoming a vehicle through which all goodness can flow through you, so that at the end of your life, you can leave the world a bit better than you found it.

I believe that we are all meant to love in our own unique way. We are also meant to connect to Love on a regular basis. I believe that all mental illness is really a disconnection from that Love. And the best way to recapture Love is to *be Love*. It's within you. I have faith in this, and I offer you all of my blessings for a peaceful joyous life where you too can unlock your Higher Self.

Afterword

It's seven in the evening on Sunday, my usual time to meet with my client Eric. I have been working with him for about ten years as a peer provider, guiding him on his journey to recovery from bipolar disorder.

When Eric came to me, he was experiencing acute bipolar symptoms, especially mania. He was living at home with his parents and in and out of the hospital. During our first session, I asked him what his goals were. He had been so beaten down by the system that he didn't want to tell me. He was tired of mental health professionals reminding him that his goals were unattainable because he had a mental illness. Yet at the end of our first session together he said, "I want to be a nurse, but it's stupid. Goodbye!" With that he ran out the door.

I didn't think I would ever see Eric again, but to my surprise, he called me to make another appointment. After some convincing, we began working towards this goal. I taught him a lot of the tools in this book.

Little by little, Eric started to make progress. Since he didn't have any education in nursing, he got his Certified Nursing Assistant certificate (CNA) and began to work in this role. He then went to nursing school. Little by little, I saw a new person start to emerge—someone who was no longer going into and out of hospitals so frequently, but someone who began to live out his life purpose.

Just as I had found for myself, once Eric felt he had a purpose, his symptoms decreased in severity, and he was able to attain his goal of becoming a nurse. He moved out of his parents' house. His life totally transformed.

Today we are having a session. Eric's progress hasn't just been on the physical plane; it's been on the spiritual one as well. Again, like me, he has found that his experience with bipolar disorder has opened him up to many of the truths in this book. Now he is not just my peer coaching client, he is a spiritual mentee who is waking up to the essence of life—that we can use our connection to something higher to transform our lives.

"Eric," I say, "I think that a lot of people do want to feel spiritually connected but get confused about how to get there. You've gotten there through reading spiritual books, prayer, meditation, and listening to my guidance as well as excellent self-care. Many people think that money, sex, alcohol, drugs, and so on are the keys to feeling as good as you are feeling. But those things in excess just blot out our Higher Power and disconnect us. Through your journey and your openness, you are waking up and experiencing the power of the Universe firsthand.

"In other societies, when people have their first break with mental illness, the community reveres them, because they know that this is the beginning of a spiritual awakening, which will turn them into healers in the community. It is scary for them, but they are immediately connected to a shaman or someone who has had a similar experience who can guide them on how to use their newfound power to help heal others. And the person inevitably does just that. I believe that peer supporters are the Western world's shamans."

"Wow," he says, excitedly, "that's actually really cool."

"Yup! It's my belief, and a belief held by many others that mental illness, along with other personal tragedies, are actually not tragedies, but windows to the Higher Self. And in our modern society, we very much need people to wake up.

"Imagine a society where everyone viewed their troubles as an opportunity to transform their lives. Half of the reason people treat each other poorly is that they believe that their troubles mean that they are not good enough or that they can't compete with others, when it's just the opposite. Obstacles are opportunities to grow and experience the abundance of life. We don't need to compete, because there is enough to go around for all of us. I think that if people truly believed this, they would not only find their happiness, but they would treat others with respect and love rather than as adversaries. This is how I believe that world peace can spread. If enough people are happy and treating others with respect, by a beautiful ripple effect we can finally experience world peace."

"Wow," Eric says, "I never thought of it like that."

"Eric," I say, "knowing this is a responsibility. I have confidence that by being a nurse and living out your mission, you will encounter other people that you can wake up too, in a way that is unique to you. Then hopefully they will do the same to others. Please don't forget this."

"I won't," he says.

And so, dear reader, I hope that I have awakened you to the very same truth through this book. We are not separate in this world, but a web of interconnected souls and energies. Once we realize this, we also realize that it is our duty not only to actualize ourselves but to pass that actualization on to others for the betterment of society.

The French Jesuit priest and paleologist Pierre Teilhard de Chardin said it best: "Someday, after mastering the winds, the waves, the tides and gravity, we shall harness for God the energies of love, and then, for a second time in the history of the world, man will have discovered fire."

My wish for you is that you take to heart the messages in this book and harness the power of Love in your own life. It is not only your birthright to overcome your own sufferings; it is your responsibility to humanity. The world needs you to fight for your wellness and find your own highest purpose and Higher Self. Each awakened spirit becomes a beacon of hope—a flame that lights other flames until the entire world and Universe are illuminated for eternity.

Resources

Here is a list of resources in the United States for people experiencing behavioral health challenges. I hope that you find them helpful. I apologize for not having a more global list, but as a US citizen, I am only recommending resources that I have interacted with or know something about.

If you are experiencing suicidal thoughts, or want to harm someone else

1. 988 Suicide and Crisis Lifeline
   Text or call 988, or chat at 988lifeline.org/

988 has been designated as the new three-digit dialing code that will route callers to the National Suicide Prevention Lifeline (now known as the 988 Suicide & Crisis Lifeline), and is active across the US.

When people call, text, or chat 988, they will be connected to trained counselors that are part of the existing Lifeline network. These trained counselors will listen, understand how their problems are affecting them, provide support, and connect them to resources if necessary.

2. The Trevor Project Crisis Line for LGBTQ Youth
   Call: 1-866-488-7386
   Text: "Start" to 678-678
   www.thetrevorproject.org/get-help/

If you are thinking about harming yourself—get immediate support. Connect to a crisis counselor 24/7, 365 days a year, from anywhere in the US. It is 100% confidential, and 100% free.

Our trained counselors understand the challenges that LGBTQ young people face. They will listen without judgment. All of your conversations are confidential, and you can share as much or as little as you'd like.

National Support Groups/Organizations For People Experiencing Behavioral Health Challenges in the United States

1. National Alliance on Mental Illness
   www.nami.org/Home

NAMI provides advocacy, education, support and public awareness so that all individuals and families affected by mental illness can build better lives.

2. Depression and Bipolar Support Alliance
www.dbsalliance.org/

DBSA offers peer-based, wellness-oriented support and empowering services. Resources are available when people need them, where they need them, and how they need to receive them—online, in local support groups, in audio and video casts, or in printed materials distributed by DBSA, our chapters, and mental health care facilities across America.

3. Hearing Voices Network
www.hearing-voices.org/

Some of the things they do:
- Share information and free resources through the website, social media, e-bulletin, newsletter, and email information service
- Engage with the media to present realistic and hopeful perspectives on hearing voices and related experiences
- Offer workshops, training and events—subject to resources
- Support members who want to set up a Hearing Voices Group

4. Mental Health America
www.mhanational.org/

MHA's programs and initiatives fulfill its mission of promoting mental health, and preventing mental illness, through advocacy, education, research and services. MHA's national office and its 200 plus affiliates and associates around the country work every day to protect the rights and dignity of individuals with lived experience and ensure that peers and their voices are integrated into all areas of the organization.

5. American Foundation for Suicide Prevention
afsp.org/

Whether you have struggled with suicide yourself or have lost a loved one, know you are not alone. Hear about personal experiences from people in your local community whose lives have been impacted by suicide.

6. Behavioral Health Resources for traditionally underrepresented communities
afsp.org/mental-health-resources-for-underrepresented
-communities#general-resources

Includes resources for the Black community, the Hispanic/ Latinx community, the Asian American community, the Native Hawaiian and Pacific Islander communities, and the Native American Community.

7. Jed Foundation
jedfoundation.org/

The Jed Foundation (JED) is a nonprofit that protects emotional health and prevents suicide for our nation's teens and young adults, giving them the skills and support they need to thrive today . . . and tomorrow.

8. National Council for Mental Wellbeing
www.thenationalcouncil.org/

Founded in 1969, the National Council for Mental Wellbeing is a membership organization that drives policy and social change on behalf of over 3,100 mental health and substance use treatment organizations, and the more than 10 million children, adults and families they serve. They advocate for policies to ensure equitable access to high-quality services. They build the capacity of mental health and substance use treatment organizations, and promote greater understanding of mental wellbeing as a core component of comprehensive health and health care. Through the Mental Health First Aid (MHFA) program, more than 2.6 million people in the US have been trained to identify, understand and respond to signs and symptoms of mental health and substance use challenges.

9. Recovery International
www.recoveryinternational.org/

Recovery International offers a cognitive behavioral training program developed by the late neuropsychiatrist Dr. Abraham Low. For more than eighty years, this method has helped people learn to identify and manage negative thoughts, feelings, beliefs, and behaviors that can lead to emotional distress and related physical symptoms. Millions of people all over the world have used this program to live more peaceful lives. Join those who have used Recovery International's self-help method to change their lives for the better.

10. Overeaters Anonymous
www.oa.org

A twelve-step community of people who through shared experience, strength, and hope are recovering from unhealthy relationships with food and body image.

11. Alcoholics Anonymous
    www.aa.org/

A twelve-step program for people who experience alcohol use disorder.

12. Recovery Dharma
    recoverydharma.org/

Recovery Dharma offers an approach to addiction recovery based on Buddhist principles. The program is peer-led and non-theistic. They welcome all those who wish to pursue recovery as part of their community.

Some Great Treatment Options/Models

1. Silver Hill Hospital
   silverhillhospital.org/

Silver Hill is an independent, not-for-profit psychiatric hospital that is nationally accredited by the independent Joint Commission. Silver Hill has been a standout among the top psychiatric hospitals in Connecticut and beyond, for adults and adolescents, since it's founding in 1931.

2. OntrackNY
   ontrackny.org/

OnTrackNY* is a mental health treatment program that empowers young people to make meaning of their experiences and to pursue their goals for school, work, and relationships.

---

* Similar models for youth experiencing a first episode of psychosis exist in other parts of the country. For one in your area look up this link: www.samhsa.gov/esmi-treatment-locator

They support the well-being of young people across New York State who are impacted by unexpected changes in their thinking and perceptions. Equity, inclusion, rapid access, and self-determination are at the core of everything they do.

3. Peer Run Crisis Respite Centers
power2u.org/directory-of-peer-respites/

Crisis Respite Centers provide an alternative to hospitalization for people experiencing emotional crises. They are warm, safe and supportive home-like places to rest and recover when more support is needed than can be provided at home.

4. Peer Support
www.samhsa.gov/brss-tacs/recovery-support-tools/peers

Peer support workers are people who have been successful in their recovery process who help others experiencing similar situations. Through shared understanding, respect, and mutual empowerment, peer support workers help people become and stay engaged in the recovery process, and reduce the likelihood of relapse. Peer support services can effectively extend the reach of treatment beyond the clinical setting into the everyday environment of those seeking a successful, sustained recovery process.

5. Become a Peer Support Specialist
copelandcenter.com/peer-specialists

This is an index with information on how to become a Peer Support Worker in Different States in the US.

Acknowledgments

It's my belief that when people give you a gift you cannot repay, the best thing to do is to pay it forward. This book was my attempt to do just that. I am so abundantly blessed by people in this lifetime so far, who have supported me in good times and bad.

To the people who made this book happen—first, Mitch Horowitz, an amazing author who saw the soul of the book before there was one and guided me in practically every part of its creation from inception all the way through connecting me to his wonderful publishing team. Thank you, Mitch; without you, there would be no *Unlocked*.

To the people at G&D Media, including Gilles Dana, Evan Litzenblatt, Ellen Goldberg, and Meghan Day Healey: you have all been a dream to work with. You've answered my endless questions as a new author, worked at lightning speed, and made this process seamless for me. Also a special thanks to

Callie Corro and Common Mode for working so hard to produce the audiobook.

To my editor, Richard Smoley: thank you for helping me take this from a manuscript to a polished book. I'm very grateful.

Deepest gratitude to my high school teacher and dear friend Marie Collins, who ignited my passion for literature and imbued me with confidence in my writing. Our relationship over the years has been the gift that keeps on giving.

To my circle of friends—thank you. There are too many of you to name, and I don't want to forget anyone, but I'll say this, if I tell you I love you, you fall into this category. Thank you for being there for me, for giving me love and time. I'm forever blessed to have you all in my life.

Thank you Emily Klein. Your ideas on our walks really helped to shape some of the major ideas in this book. Love you.

Thanks to my extended family—The Pomerantz clan, cousins Amy and Susan Wilson, and my brother Matt Freeman—I'm lucky to call you my family—your support and acceptance of me over the years has been tremendous. Love you all very much.

To my family friends who are family, including the Franzblaus, Laskys, and Borshoffs thank you for always loving me exactly as I am, and standing by me no matter what. I inherited you all as friends because I have wonderful parents who know how to be great friends—what a blessing you all are to me.

To Elaine Franzblau, who has been such a true-blue friend since I was born: I cannot express how much I love you or how grateful I am to have a friend like you. You stood by me during the worst of times, and you've celebrated with me during the best of times. I'm so blessed by you, and so glad my mom knows how to share friends.

Infinite gratitude to my Buddhist community, especially Gonzalo Obelleiro, and my dear ones in the Montclair South District, including our fearless leader and my dear friend Glenda Rich. Growing with all of you has been a privilege, and I know that I wouldn't have had the confidence to publish this without you. To Bonnie Reed, Carolyn Somerville, and Beth Popper—your hours of guidance have been invaluable, and much of your wisdom is infused in this book.

To Daisaku Ikeda—without your fearlessness in bringing our practice to America from Japan, I would have never heard the words *nam myoho renge kyo*. I have a deep debt of gratitude to you.

I'm so lucky to also have had some incredible career mentors. Infinite thanks to all of the people who have believed in me and supported my career, including Dr. Edye Schwartz, Mark Graham, LCSW, Dr. Patricia Deegan, Dr. Jorge Petit, Dr. Alec Miller, Dr. Amy Spagnolo, and Dr. Carlos Pratt. Your guidance has been tremendous, and I wouldn't be where I am today without all of you. As they say, I'm standing on the shoulders of giants!

Thanks to all of the sponsors and friends in the Overeaters Anonymous community. While I will keep you all anonymous, I'm nonetheless extremely grateful for all of your time and love. I'm better for having all of you in my life.

To my beautiful, witchy sister, Pam Grossman: your advice at critical moments and turning points in the publishing process has been invaluable. I love you, and I'm so grateful to be your sister.

To Sherrie Schwab, therapist extraordinaire, and one of my biggest cheerleaders in my darkest time: there are no words to describe what you did and how you changed my life with your therapeutic style and wisdom. Thank you for sticking with me when others had given up on me and reminding me that there was a "well" version of me inside of me all along.

Deep gratitude to my "bestie" Shannon Hivick, who was the first to read my manuscript and who continually encouraged me to publish in the first place. I'm so grateful that you were born and that you came into my life when you did.

Finally, to my parents, Nina and Richard Grossman: when you start life on third base trying to run home with the kind of parents I have in you both, you *owe* it back to the world to help others. Most people don't have parents like you. I know that I wouldn't be recovered without the undying love and support of you both. The wisdom that is infused in this book is full of lessons learned from both of you. I love you infinitely.

A note about names: a number of names in this book have been changed to protect confidentiality.

About the Author

Emily Grossman, MA, CPRP, NYCPS-P is a Peer Specialist, keynote speaker, trainer, and writer with fifteen years of experience working in the mental health field.

Emily speaks nationally about her miraculous mental health recovery journey, and her belief that recovery should be expected for people with behavioral health challenges. She is proud to be hospital free and living in recovery from bipolar disorder for the last fifteen years.

In addition to this work, she is the Director of the Training Institute at Coordinated Behavioral Care, Inc, a mental health non-profit in NYC. In this role, she coordinates training and trains mental health professionals across New York State.

Emily has also written for Huffington Post about her own recovery from bipolar disorder. She is a Certified Psychiatric Rehabilitation Practitioner and has a Master's in Education from Columbia University's Teachers College.

In 2018, Emily was named "Peer Specialist of The Year" by the National Council for Mental Wellbeing.

While Emily brings years of experience both personally and professionally to each audience she speaks with, she also brings her heart.

For more information on Emily and her mission, please visit www.emilygrossman.net.

CPSIA information can be obtained
at www.ICGtesting.com
Printed in the USA
JSHW052029290623
43772JS00005B/5

9 781722 506520